Introduction *to* Medicinal Cannabis

Introduction *to* Medicinal Cannabis

A Practical Guide for Health Professionals & Patients

Dr Teresa Towpik

Table of Contents

"

Marijuana in its natural form is one of the safest thera-
peutically active substances known to man. By any measure of
rational analysis marijuana can be safely used within the super-
vised routine of medical care.

Francis Young

US Drug Enforcement Administration Chief
Administrative Law Judge – 1988

Acknowledgements

I would like to acknowledge the key people who played criti-cal roles in the production of this book. Thank you to Mariusz Krzeszewski, Pavel Bulkiewicz, Luka Bankovic as well as Warwick Stanley for their help with editing and attention to detail.

I would also like to acknowledge all of the people who kindly agreed to read this book and provided me with constructive and valuable feedback.

Preface

Welcome to the second edition of Introduction to Medicinal Cannabis.

It has been quite the journey since the first edition in December 2017.

As my learning process continues and my fascination with the cannabis plant grows, I am witness to the many gifts it has to offer to my patients.

To my new readers, I will introduce myself as a GP who studied medicine in Poland, my country of birth, before beginning my career in Australia in 1993.

As a conventional doctor I have practised evidence-based medicine and followed the guidelines diligently. I still do.

At the same time, I've always felt there is much more to healing than simply prescribing pills. As well as wanting to go deeper into why we get sick in first place, I felt a need to learn more about plants and herbs and practise more holistically.

I researched and learnt about various methods. My experience with breast cancer in 2001 showed me that healing can occur on multiple levels: physical, emotional, mental and spiritual. I believe the healing process is personal and unique for each person.

As a traditional GP, I held biased and limited views regarding cannabis. I felt it was illegal for valid reasons, being highly addictive, harmful and a gateway to heavier drugs such as heroin.

I had not been aware of therapeutic properties of cannabis until January 2016 when I heard that the nation's laws were going to be amended legalising it for medicinal use.

This news came as a revelation to me. I felt perhaps it could be the answer to my hopes of introducing a more holistic and natural approach to my practice.

As I began researching cannabis, I quickly realised how

mistaken I had been in my attitude, which had lacked any base of knowledge and understanding.

While studying the plant and its history, I heard people talking about their experiences with medicinal cannabis and was touched and inspired by their stories.

Perhaps the most amazing were the stories of children suffering from intractable epilepsy, who were going through 50-100 seizures per day. They were not responding to conventional drugs and they were experiencing many adverse effects. For many of them cannabis brought life-changing improvements.

I decided to get actively involved in promoting cannabis treatments and educating the general public – and to hopefully interest other GPs who may be sceptical and dismissive of it, as I once was.

In researching cannabis and its therapeutic properties, my initial learning experience was chaotic and frustrating. I struggled with so much information online and was searching for more structured education for busy doctors. With that in mind I funded MediHuanna in October 2016.

MediHuanna is devoted to educating health professionals about the science of medicinal cannabis and equipping them with the practical skills necessary to treat and prescribe for patients who would benefit from its use.

Our online and face-to-face courses have received accreditation from the Royal College of General Practitioners (RACGP), the professional body of GPs responsible for maintaining the standards of GP education.

I have been prescribing cannabis since March 2018. I feel extremely privileged to witness many life-changing experiences among my patients. Being able to guide them and see them getting better is very rewarding.

To those who had not yet read or heard of this book's first edi-tion, this its extended version, adding testimonials from grateful patients and including full referencing of the book's information.

In this edition, I share some of my clinical experience in using medicinal cannabis in general practice. I have also added chapters on patient care, dosing, management and monitoring.

It is a comprehensive, practical introduction to cannabis medi-cine for health professionals and could also be useful for patients wanting to learn about it.

I hope to inspire my fellow doctors to learn about the remark-able properties of this plant and to embrace it as an important therapeutic agent that will widen their treatment options.

My personal experience in prescribing cannabis in Australia

Cannabis was legalised in Australia for medicinal use in January 2016 but at that time it was almost impossible for any GP to obtain approval through existing legal channels. I had to fight for more than eight months to obtain an approval for one of my patients. The process was difficult, convoluted and riddled with red tape, requiring hours of paperwork and perseverance – a thoroughly discouraging undertaking for busy doctors.

One of the major obstacles was the need for GP's to obtain the endorsement from the specialist. Unfortunately, the majority of specialists I had contacted were opposed to using cannabis. They would argue lack of evidence and proper randomised clinical trials, addiction potential concerns, unknown long-term effects and so on. Many of these views were based on fear, dogma and lack of education about cannabis as a therapeutical agent.

Fortunately, since mid-March 2018, the process of prescribing cannabis, although not ideal, is much improved and simplified. I hope to see a time when it will be a matter of writing a script and sending the patient to a local chemist.

At the time of writing this chapter (March 2019), I have obtained approval for 82 patients within the last 12 months. My main focus is chronic debilitating pain that is unresponsive to conventional pharmaceuticals. I applied through SAS cat B and from October 2018 through the Authorised Prescriber scheme. Within that group, I had 43 females and 39 males, ages ranging from 21 to 93, with the majority over 50 years-old. Thirty-eight per cent of patients related their pain to past injury. These statistics appear to correlate with general available data on prescribing of medicinal cannabis.

Seventy-one of my patients suffered from chronic non-cancer

pain secondary to multiple conditions, in particular lumbar and cervical spondylosis, arthritis, migraine, fibromyalgia, protracted post-surgical pain and many others, including multiple sclerosis.

The chronic pain cases were accompanied by multiple comorbidities, such as PTSD, anxiety, depression, insomnia, high cholesterol, hypertension, ischaemic heart disease, diabetes, atrial fibrillation, obesity, gastro-oesophageal reflux, bi-polar disorder, gout, pulmonary fibrosis, COPD and asthma.

Eight patients presented with cancer-related pain and within that group, four passed away. They did, however, experience the benefits of cannabis such as improved overall quality of life, better mood, sleep, appetite and noticeable declines in the frequency of nausea, vomiting and pain.

Most importantly, cannabis allowed these patients to interact with their loved ones in the way they had previously enjoyed. They were able to use less of the conventional drugs, in particular opioids, and their families in turn were grateful their loved ones passed away peacefully.

Among my current patients who have responded well to treatment is one who presented with schizoaffective disorder accompanied by PTSD, insomnia and debilitating anxiety. He was prescribed pure CBD oil, which proved to be safer and more effective than conventionally prescribed anti-psychotics and with no adverse effects.

Not all treatments were successful. In the cases of one patient suffering from epilepsy and another who suffered from both autism and epilepsy, I prescribed low THC and high CBD formulation, which seemed to aggravate their symptoms. However, the circumstances were quite complex and difficult. I believe that with easy access to a variety of affordable cannabis products, and the availability of varying ratios of cannabinoids, terpenes and flavonoids, we would be able to find the right formulations for this category of patient.

For the most part, the adverse effects I have observed were rather mild. Drowsiness, for example, was mitigated by taking cannabis at night. Some patients complained of fatigue, however, other benefits, in particular pain relief, outweighed this issue. A few patients complained of agitation, dry mouth and increased appetite, which eventually subsided as the treatment continued.

The most common reason for halting cannabis treatment was the excessive cost, at around $200 to $500 per month. The majority of my patients are low-income earners, health-care card holders or pensioners. Unfortunately, they fall within the demographic who need this treatment most but often can't afford it.

Three of my patients experienced an episode of psychoactive effects. Two of them were managed successfully by stopping their medicine for 3-4 nights and restarting at a previously tolerated dose. The third patient found this experience too difficult to tolerate. She decided to discontinue, especially that her response to cannabis treatment had been rather subtle and she could not justify the ongoing expense.

In the relatively short period of time I have been prescribing cannabis – and among the relatively small number of patients - I have already witnessed a large percentile of impressive beneficial responses.

Some of the observed patterns and benefits included:

- Superior safety profile in comparison to my experience with the majority of conventional pharmaceuticals.
- Ability to help many clinical conditions patients may suffer from. For example, I observed beneficial effects on other comorbidities such as skin problems, gut symptoms, diabetes, depression, anxiety and PTSD. I feel confident now that cannabis can be used to treat multiple symptoms

and medical conditions simultaneously.
- Improved functionality. Patients started socialising more, going to the gym, and generally being able to accomplish more during the day.
- Some of my grossly obese patients managed to lose a lot of weight, between 10-20 kg, which they had previously found impossible to achieve.
- Improved overall quality of life.
- Improved ability to focus, motivate and concentrate. I was quite surprised to hear the comment, "my mind is not so foggy any more".
- Varying degrees of pain reduction, modest for some and quite significant for others, including a group who experienced previously uncommon periods of no pain.
- About 50 per cent of my patients were able to reduce or even stop their other medications, in particular opioids.
- About 80-90 per cent reported improved sleep.
- No escalation in doses nor drug seeking behaviours.

I have used various cannabis oil formulations which included pure CBD, low THC-high CBD and equal THC to CBD products administered orally. In my experience, balanced cannabinoid formulations with equal amounts of THC and CBD are most effective in the treatment of chronic pain and allow smaller volumes to be used, making it more affordable for the patients.

Cannabis offers the possibility of substantial cost savings to the health-care system. By effectively treating the community, we can reduce the number of avoidable hospital admissions and interventional procedures, such as cardiac procedures, joint replacements and so on. The need for polypharmacy could be reduced, since cannabis can be used to treat many conditions at the same time. Patients observe improved functionality, in turn providing those unable to work with better chances of returning to the workforce and thus reducing reliance on welfare benefits.

I feel very fortunate and privileged to be able to prescribe cannabis and witness life-changing situations for many of my patients. I believe cannabis is a safe and effective treatment option for patients suffering from chronic pain as well as many other clinical conditions. I hope it will become more affordable and accessible for those who need it most and that more doctors will embrace it as an important therapeutic agent.

My vision and dream is to see cannabis integrated into modern medicine along with other modalities of healing in a multidisciplinary and holistic model of care.

For health professionals interested in learning about current process in Australia, please visit our website **www.medihuanna.com** to obtain information about our RACGP-accredited courses for doctors.

The Basics

The History of Cannabis

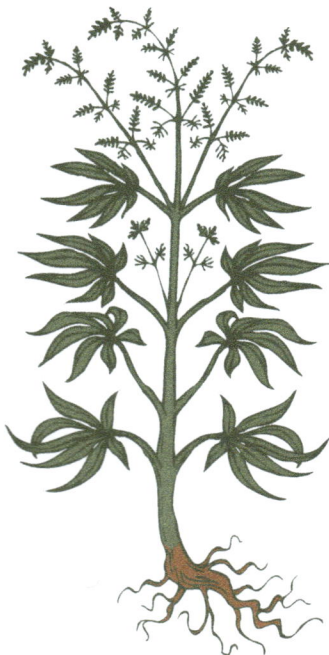

Cannabis has been assisting humans for thousands of years. As one of the first domesticated crops it was used as medicine, food, textile, rope, fish-nets and as a part of spiritual and sacramental practices, with shamans and mystics using it as a means to communicate with the divine.

The cannabis plant is believed to have come to human attention about 12,000 years ago in Central Asia. It was introduced to western medicine in 1841 by a famous Irish physician, Sir William O'Shaughnessy, upon his return from British India.[1] While there, O'Shaughnessy researched cannabis and made many cannabis preparations, initially testing them on animals. Later, after establishing their safety, he used them on humans and found them useful in the treatment of rabies, cholera, tetanus and infantile convulsions.

Cannabis was used extensively in the forms of tinctures, pills and extracts until its 20th century prohibition. It was even a part of cough mixtures for children. Queen Victoria used cannabis in the treatment of menstrual cramps. It was prescribed by doctors and prepared by pharmacists. In 1915, famous English physician, Sir William Osler, referred to cannabis as perhaps the best remedy for severe headaches, especially migraines.

Today's major pharmaceutical companies were some of the original sellers of cannabis. These include Eli Lilly, Parke-Davis (now owned by Pfizer) and Squibb of Bristol-Myers Squibb. Medical marijuana was a huge seller at the turn of the century.

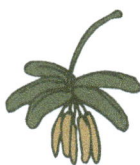

Smoking of cannabis was unknown in developed countries apart from its occasional use in the treatment of asthma. Recreational cannabis smoking became popular in the US after 1910, during an influx of Mexican migrants.

In the early 1920s, several countries, including Mexico, South Africa and Canada, banned cannabis, signalling the beginning of the end of its close relationship with humankind. By 1925, it had been added to the list of drugs prohibited under the League of Nations' revised International Opium Convention. The Commissioner of the US Treasury Department Bureau of Narcotics, Harry Anslinger, later succeeded in directing both the League of Nations and its successor, the United Nations, to ban cannabis worldwide.

Cannabis was included in the US Pharmacopoeia until 1942 but its branding by Anslinger as "killer weed", "assassin of youth" and a "gateway drug" had swayed authorities against it.

The world is now aware that cannabis prohibition was a sop to the vested interests of political and business lobbies and had nothing to do with the pharmacological properties of the plant. In fact, the then president of American Medical Association, Dr William Woodward, opposed prohibition, claiming it would stagnate the medicinal use and the scientific research of the plant.

One of the contributing factors to its removal from the US pharmacopoeia register was the advent of single-molecule synthetic drugs. Major pharmaceutical companies began introducing them at the beginning of the 20th century as a reputedly more effective, safe and predictable medicine. They were considered easier to research, patent and sell. Doctors were trained to trust these formulations and to look down at herbal medicine as inferior, unpredictable and basically something of a tonic or placebo.

Cannabis never disappeared, of course, but simply went

"underground" - and now, after decades of prohibition for all the wrong reasons, much of the western world is experiencing a cannabis renaissance.

I believe that because of prohibition we have missed out on a lot of scientific research and knowledge around the medicinal use of cannabis. Prohibition led to the creation of the black market, which focused mostly on the narcotic effects of the plant and drove production of high-THC cannabis strains.

In spite of prohibition, some scientific discoveries were still occurring. In 1964 Israeli organic chemist Raphael Mechoulam isolated THC, delta-9-tetrahydeocannabinol, the most famous ingredient in the cannabis plant and best known for its psychoactive effects. However, the psychoactive properties of THC are just part of the story. This molecule is highly therapeutic, as will be explained in following chapters.

The discovery of THC opened the doors to further research and a better understanding of human physiology. In the years following the finding, hundreds of other cannabinoids were discovered. The most widely known, cannabidiol, or CBD, was first isolated by Roger Adams in 1940 and its molecular structure was elucidated by Prof. Mechoulam and his team in 1963. CBD is the second-most abundant, and non-addictive component of the cannabis plant and is characterised by a very low level of toxicity. The 1990s saw the cloning of CB1 and CB2 receptors, followed by the discovery of our own endocannabinoids, anandamide and 2-AG. Finally, the Endocannabinoid System was discovered. It is the universal system of internal regulation, cellular communication and homeostasis, present in humans, animals and plants.

What we are observing now in the cannabis space is fascinating, and our increasing knowledge and acceptance of the plant's properties is moving around the world like a tsunami. Medicinal use of cannabis is widely accepted by the general public while continuing to divide the medical profession and policymakers. I believe we need to let go of the attitude of fear and the dogma surrounding this important plant and start educating ourselves about its benefits.

The Cannabis Plant

There are thousands of different cannabis species called **chemovars** (commonly referred to as strains). Each chemovar contains various combinations of **cannabinoids, terpenes** and **flavonoids**. These components possess important **pharmacological and modulatory properties**. The three main cannabis species are Cannabis Indica Cannabis Sativa (industrial hemp belongs here) and Cannabis Ruderalis

Cannabis Indica

PROPERTIES

Cannabis Indica has relaxing and calming effects, therefore is best suited for night use. The sedative effect of the most common cannabis strains is attributable to their **myrcene content**, a mono-terpene known for its sedative **couch-lock effect**.[2,3]

THE LOOK

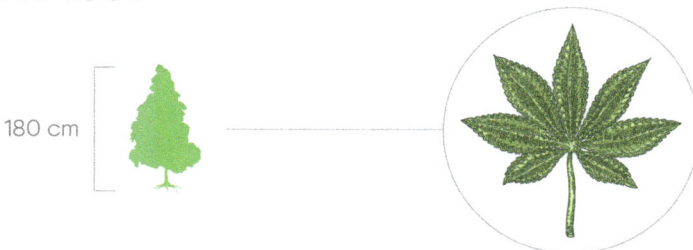

180 cm

Indica is short, wide and bushy. It has broad and thick leaves.[2]

Cannabis Sativa

PROPERTIES

Cannabis sativa is uplifting, energetic, cerebral, hallucinogenic and best suited to day use.[2]

THE LOOK

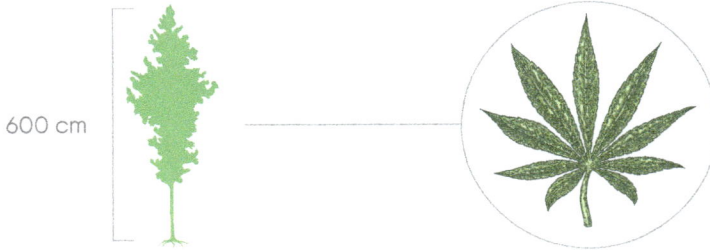

600 cm

Sativa plants are tall, growing up to six metres, and have slender, spiky leaves.[2]

Cannabis Ruderalis – "the rugged weed"

PROPERTIES

Cannabis ruderalis is a low-THC species of cannabis native to Central and Eastern Europe and Russia.[4]

THE LOOK

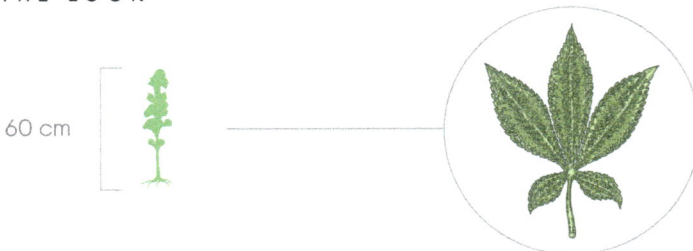

60 cm

It is short, rarely growing over 60 cm in height and is characterised by a fibrous stem with small amounts of branches growing from it.[3] It's a hardy plant and tolerates cold climate well.

The active ingredients in all these species are **cannabinoids, terpenes** and **flavonoids**.[5]

Endocannabinoid System (ECS)

The endocannabinoid system, named after the plant that led to its discovery, is the universal, omnipresent system of internal regulation, cellular communication and homeostasis. It plays an important role in establishing and maintaining human health. It is present in humans, animals and plants alike, except insects. It is believed this system appeared about 500 million years ago and kept evolving.[6]

The discovery of this system is a result of significant research since 1964. In that year, famous Israeli scientist Professor Mechoulam and his team isolated THC, Δ^9-Tetrahydrocannabinol, the most abundant part of cannabis responsible for its psychoactive effects: the feelings of euphoria and sedation.[7]

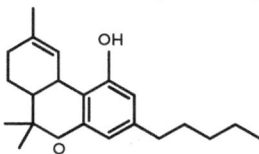

Δ^9-Tetrahydrocannabinol
(THC)

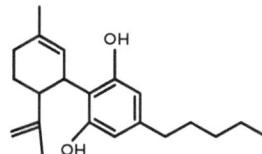

Cannabidiol (CBD)

The now famous CBD (cannabidiol), was first obtained from the cannabis plant in 1940 by Roger Adams and his colleagues. Its molecular structure was then elucidated by Prof. Mechoulam and his team in 1963[8]. In comparison to THC, CBD is the second-most abundant, non-psychoactive, non-addictive part of the cannabis plant, and as previously outlined, characterised by its low level of toxicity.[9]

The isolation of THC opened the doors to a better understanding of how our body and brain function and further research led to the isolation of hundreds of other cannabinoids. In the 1990s, researchers cloned cannabinoid receptors that are present throughout the human body. These are CB1 receptors, mostly found in the central nervous system, and the CB2 receptors mostly found in the immune system and its associated structures.[7]

Following the discoveries of exogenous plant cannabinoids, scientists isolated endogenous cannabinoids also known as endocannabinoids: anandamide and 2-AG. These molecules are naturally produced in the human body. Both endocannabinoids and THC are similar in molecular structure and interact with cannabinoid receptors, based on the key and lock analogy.[6]

The endocannabinoid system consists of three major components.[6,7,10]

- The cannabinoid receptors: **CB1** and **CB2**
- The endocannabinoids that interact with these receptors: **anandamide** and **2-AG**.
- The **enzymes** which are involved in the synthesis and degradation of these endocannabinoids. The ones responsible for degradation are **Fatty Acid Amide Hydrolase (FAAH)** and **Monoacylglycerol Lipase (MAGL)**

This system is involved in the regulation of many physiological processes including [6]:

- Stress
- Emotion
- Memory
- Cognition
- Sleep

- Digestion
- Inflammation
- Thermoregulation
- Neural development
- Neuroprotection
- Movement
- Psychomotor behaviour
- Pain
- Cardiovascular and immune function
- Metabolism
- Appetite regulation

In short, the role of the endocannabinoid system can be described as controlling eat, sleep, relax, forget and protect functions[11]. These basic functions of the ECS were summarised in 1998 by Professor Di Marzo.

It is very interesting that the endocannabinoid system was unravelled more than 20 years ago in what is now considered by some as the most important discovery of the 20th century in human biology. However, sadly the majority of health professionals, including myself until three years ago, were unaware of this important system. It has not been part of the curriculum in medical schools.

Cannabinoid Receptors

Cannabinoid receptors belong to the family of G protein-coupled receptors (GPCRs). Both receptors are located in the presynaptic neurons and play an important role in modulating neurotransmitters release.[6,7,10] These are CB1 and CB2 receptors.

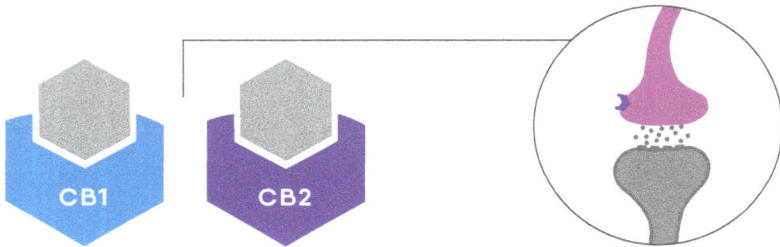

Both receptors are located in the presynaptic neurons and play an important role in modulating neurotransmitters release.

THC acts like a key that unlocks both receptors, mediating most of its psychoactive effects by interacting with CB1 receptors in the brain.[12]

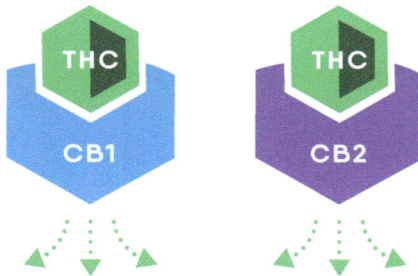

THC acts as a partial agonist at CB1 and CB2 receptors

Furthermore, THC molecule acts as a partial agonist at both CB1 and CB2 receptors.[13]

CB1 Receptor

The CB1 receptors are primarily found in the nervous system, mostly in the brain and spinal cord. Our brains are densely populated by these receptors, especially the cerebellum, hippocampus, amygdala, basal ganglia and frontal cortex.[6,10,12] The presence of CB1 receptors in these parts of the brain indicates their involvement in memory, cognition, emotions, movement and nociception.[14]

CB1 receptors are one of the most abundant G protein-coupled receptors (GPCRs) in the central nervous system (CNS).[12] Furthermore, they are 10 times more common in the brain than opioid receptors.[6]

The low densities of CB1 receptors in the brainstem, especially **cardiorespiratory centres**, which are responsible for maintaining vital life functions, might explain why there are no reported cases of lethal cannabis overdose.[6]

CB1 receptors are also found on peripheral nerve terminals as well as peripheral tissues[15] within a group including testes, uterus, adipose and connective tissues, endocrine and exocrine glands, leucocytes, spleen, liver and the gastrointestinal tract.

CB2 Receptor

The CB2 receptors are mostly found in the immune system, which implies the possibility that the endocannabinoid system has an immuno-modulatory role. When these receptors are activated, the physiological effects often tend to be beneficial, for example in reducing inflammation.[16]

CB2 receptors are prominent in peripheral tissues, including:

- Monocytes,
- Macrophages,
- B-cells, T-cells,

- Liver, Spleen, Tonsils,
- CNS and the Enteric nervous system.[17]

Although less predominate, CB2 receptors are also found throughout the CNS and are located on primary sensory neurons and microglial cells.[6,12] In the CNS, the expression of these receptors is associated with inflammation.[12]

Scientists believe that CB2 receptors are involved in the pharmacological effects of cannabinoids on inflammation and immunological function.[6] CB2 expression is amplified by inflammation, which suggests these receptors may be involved in the endogenous response to injury.[6]

Endogenous Cannabinoids

I find it fascinating that our own bodies produce cannabinoids naturally similar to THC. These internally produced molecules are known as endogenous cannabinoids or endocannabinoids. To date, the two well-established endocannabinoids include: N-Arachidonoylethanolamine (Anandamide) and 2-Arachidonoylglycerol (2-AG).[6,10]

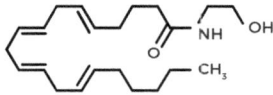

N-Arachidonoylethanolamine
(Anandamide or AEA)

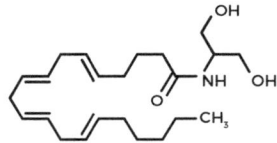

2-Arachidonoylglycerol (2-AG)

Anandamide, often referred to as the 'bliss molecule' is named after the Sanskrit word Ananda, meaning supreme joy, bliss or happiness. This molecule binds to both cannabinoid receptors as **partial agonist**. It has moderately higher affinity to CB1 receptors.[6,10,18] **2-AG** has been found present in the brain at concentrations 170 times greater than Anandamide and binds to both CB1 and CB2 receptors as **full agonist**.[19]

Both Anandamide and 2-AG are retrograde messengers in the nervous system, **synthesised on demand** and are characterised by a **short half-life**. Therefore, the body will only produce them when needed.[20]Endocannabinoids, being lipids, are not stored like other neurotransmitters. Their concentrations increase with stimulation, leading to the concept that they are **deployed when required**.[21]

Once released from the post-synaptic neuron, they travel back to the presynaptic neuron and bind to the cannabinoid receptors. Then they are promptly degraded by the enzymes, fatty acid amide hydrolase (FAAH) and monoacylglycerol lipase (MAGL).[20]

To summarise, both endogenous cannabinoids possess the following characteristics.[22]

- Crucial role in bio-regulation
- Main role in cell-signalling
- Lipid structure, making them lipophilic
- Hydrophobic
- Local cell-signalling (paracrine or autocrine)
- Retrograde transmission in the brain
- Formed from the internal lipid constituents on cellular membrane
- Synthesised on demand and not stored
- Very short half-life
- Degradation by FAAH and MAGL may regulate ECS bioactivity

Key and Lock Analogy

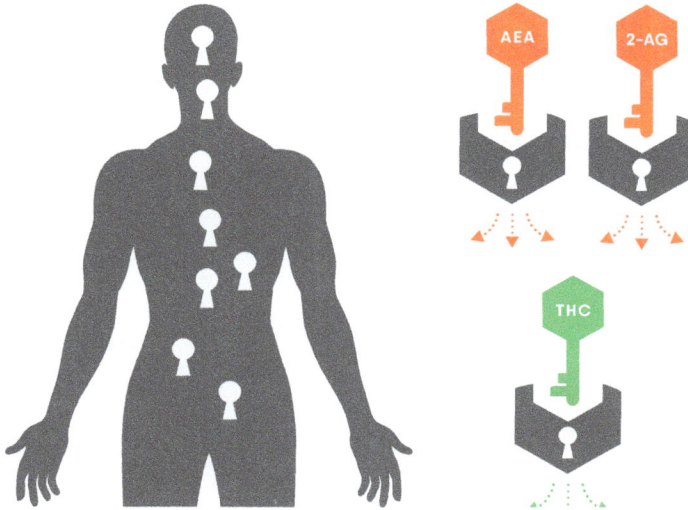

Cannabinoids are the key, while receptors are the lock.

Both endogenous and exogenous cannabinoids interact with CB1 and CB2 receptors based on the **key and lock analogy**. In this mechanism, cannabinoids are the key, while receptors, which are located in the cell membranes, are the lock.[23]

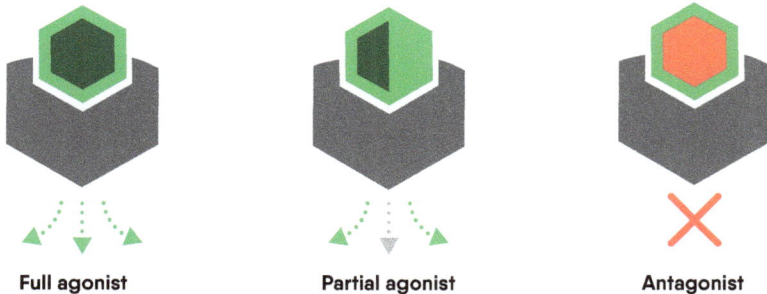

Full agonist   Partial agonist   Antagonist

Cannabinoids can behave as agonists or antagonists. In general, if a particular molecule binds to the receptor causing it to start a physiological action, it is defined as **agonist**. If that molecule binds to a receptor and blocks the physiological action, it is defined as **antagonist**.[24]

Taking the key and lock metaphor a bit further, sometimes, when we put a key in the lock, it fits and we can turn it to open the door either fully (**full agonist**) or partially (**partial agonist**). However, sometimes, when we put a key in a lock, it fits but we are unable to turn it to open the door. This metaphor describes **antagonist**.

Allosteric and Orthosteric receptor binding site

Orthosteric is the active site of the receptor, the key and lock analogy site. **Allosteric** is the site where ligands (molecules) bind elsewhere on the receptor surface, and allosterically change the conformation of the receptor binding site.[25]

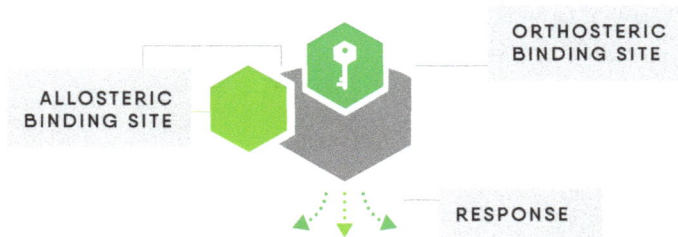

Both endogenous and exogenous cannabinoids, including THC, bind to the orthosteric receptor site.[26] CBD binds weakly to allosteric site as a negative allosteric modulator.[27]

The Endocannabinoid System in Action

The endocannabinoid system plays an important role in maintaining homeostasis in our bodies. Below is a simplified, step by step explanation of how the endocannabinoid system works in the neuron and how it regulates neurotransmitter release in our bodies.

1. Neurons communicate with each other through electrochemical impulses. The electrical impulse, known as **action potential**, travels down the presynaptic neuron.[28]

2. This action triggers many processes and among them the **opening of the calcium channels**.

3. Calcium influx causes the **release of neurotransmitters** stored in presynaptic vesicles.[28]

4. These neurotransmitters travel across the **synaptic cleft** and bind to the **receptors in the postsynaptic neuron.**

5. If everything is in balance and the body maintains homeostasis, the process will be repeated and the message continues to spread across the neurons. However, if the neurotransmitters are upregulated with too much inhibition or excitation, calcium channels in the postsynaptic neuron will open up.[29,30]

6. The calcium influx leads to the synthesis of endocannabinoids, **Anandamide (AEA)** and **2-AG**. These endocannabinoids are produced in the cellular membrane of the postsynaptic neuron and travel back to the presynaptic neuron.[29,30]

ECS in action

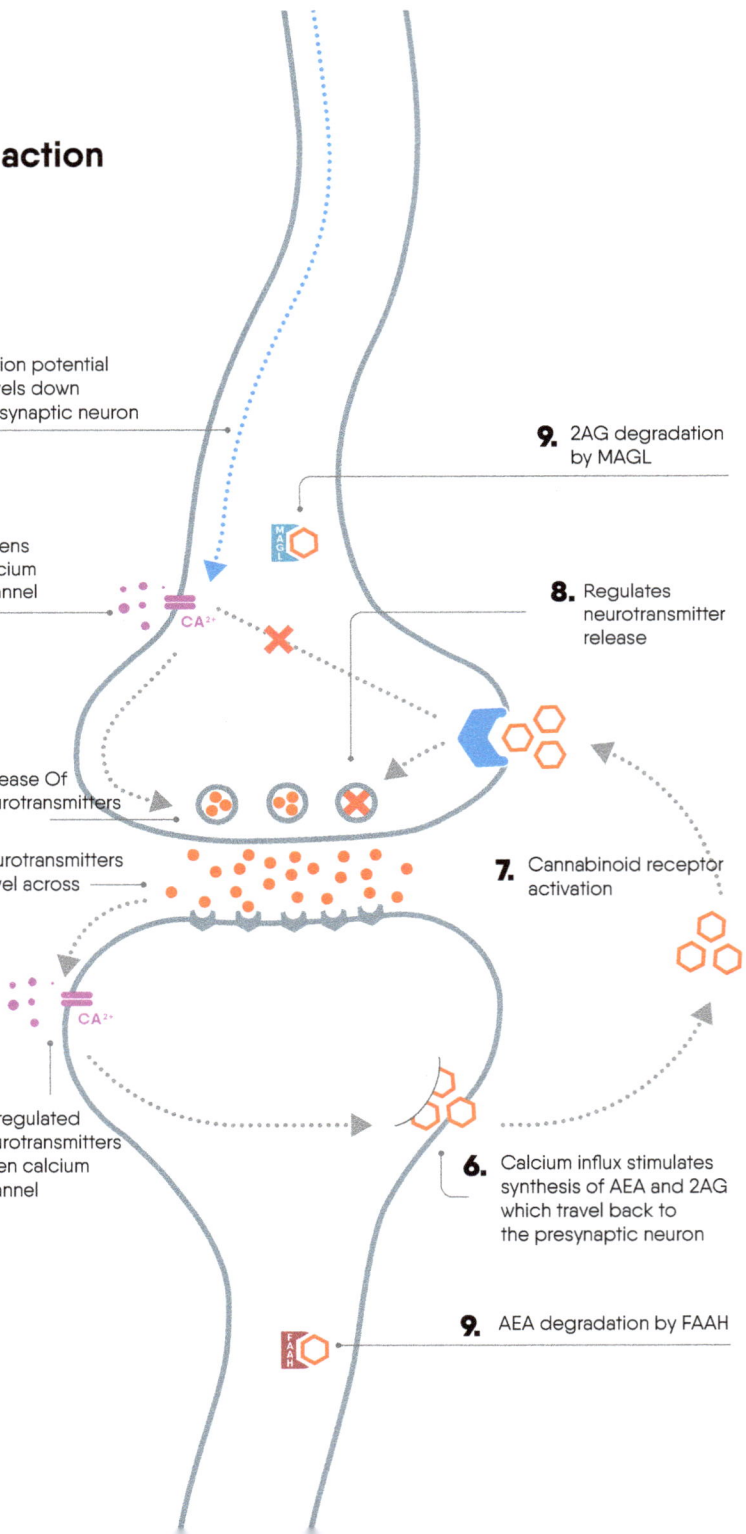

1. Action potential travels down presynaptic neuron

2. Opens calcium channel

CA²⁺

3. Release Of neurotransmitters

4. Neurotransmitters travel across

5. Upregulated neurotransmitters open calcium channel

CA²⁺

6. Calcium influx stimulates synthesis of AEA and 2AG which travel back to the presynaptic neuron

7. Cannabinoid receptor activation

8. Regulates neurotransmitter release

9. 2AG degradation by MAGL

MAGL

9. AEA degradation by FAAH

FAAH

7. Anandamide and 2-AG activate cannabinoid receptors in the presynaptic neuron.[19] This process is known as **retrograde signalling**, where these endocannabinoids serve as retrograde messengers communicating with the cannabinoid receptors.

8. **Activation of the CB1 receptor** causes the **closing of the calcium channel** in the pre-synaptic neuron and regulates further release of neurotransmitters.

9. Once this process is completed, these endocannabinoids are quickly eliminated. Recent studies indicate the presence of intracellular transporters known as **Fatty Acid Binding Proteins (FABP)** which are taking these molecules to their **degradation site**.[20] 2-AG is transported to its degradation site in the presynaptic neuron and is metabolised by the enzyme **MAGL**. Anandamide is transported to its degradation site in the postsynaptic neuron and is metabolised by the enzyme **FAAH**.[29]

In summary, the endocannabinoid system is essential in maintaining balance in human body. It works like a thermostat that regulates the release of neurotransmitters. The overall process is far more complicated. This is just a simple explanation of the endocannabinoid system in action to convey its core functions.

Pharmacology

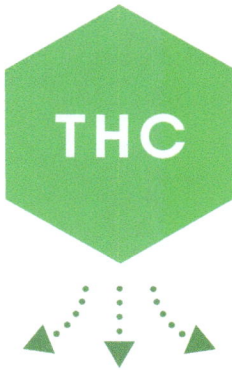

Delta 9-Tetrahydrocannabinol (THC)

Δ^9-Tetrahydrocannabinol (THC) is the main psychoactive component in the cannabis plant. It is produced within the **glandular trichomes**, the highest concentration of which are on the flowers of the unfertilised female plant.[1]

THC interacts with the human body by activating CB1 and CB2 cannabinoid receptors.[2,3] It is a **weak partial agonist** to these receptors.[4] Psychoactive effects of THC are the result of activation of CB1 receptors in the brain.[2,4] This activation may trigger various responses in the following parts of the brain:

- **Amygdala** - Panic and paranoia
- **Basal ganglia** - Slowed reaction time
- **Brain stem** - Antiemetic effects
- **Cerebellum** - Impaired coordination
- **Hippocampus** - Impaired memory
- **Hypothalamus** - Increased appetite or "munchies"
- **Neocortex** - Altered thinking, judgment and sensation
- **Nucleus accumbens** - Euphoria, or sense of wellness and feeling good
- **Spinal cord** - Altered pain sensation[5]

Although more research is needed, THC is emerging to be an important therapeutic agent with a wide range of medicinal properties, which include:

- **Analgesia** due to activation of CB1 and CB2 receptors at the level of peripheral nerves, spinal cord and brain[4]
- Possible **anti-inflammatory functions** through activation of the CB1 and CB2 receptors[6] as well as many other

contributions.[4] It has twenty times the anti-inflammatory potency of aspirin and twice that of hydrocortisone[7]

- **Anti-Nausea** and **anti-vomiting** due to activation of CB1 receptors in the brain stem[8,9]
- **Appetite stimulation** as a result of activation of CB1 receptors in the hypothalamus[10]
- **Anti-convulsant** due to an apparent apposite quality that regulates neuronal excitability during seizures. However, this characteristic requires more research before it can be positively identified as having the potential to **control seizures.**[11]
- **Anti-cancer** properties that may inhibit tumour growth and angiogenesis.[12]
- **Antioxidant** properties in both THC and CBD[13] which are more potent antioxidants than vitamins C and E.[2]

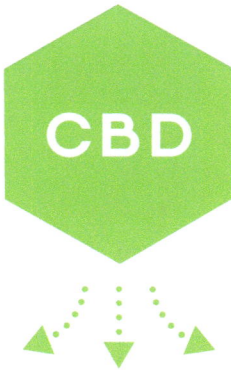

Cannabidiol (CBD)

Cannabidiol (CBD) is the second most abundant, non-psychoactive and non-addictive part of the cannabis plant.[14] It binds very weakly to CB1 and CB2 receptors on the allosteric binding site.[15] Characterised by its very low toxicity, it exerts therapeutic effects by interacting with multiple metabolic pathways in the human body.

- **CBD modulates the psychoactive effects of THC**. Recent evidence suggests it may be a negative allosteric modulator of the CB1 receptor, thereby acting as a non-competitive antagonist of the actions of THC and other CB1 agonists.[14] CBD inhibits fatty acid amide hydrolase (FAAH), thus increasing anandamide (AEA) levels and making CB1 receptors occupied for longer periods of time and preventing THC from binding to them.[16]

- **Analgesic effects**. CBD may exert its analgesic effects by interacting agonistically with the **TRPV1** receptor, which is known to mediate pain perception, inflammation and body temperature.[17] CBD also interacts with the **glycine receptors** which mediate neuropathic pain and inflammation.[14,18,19]

- **Anxiolytic and antidepressant**. CBD may exert anxiolytic and antidepressant properties through agonistic interaction with adenosine receptors. Activation of these receptors downregulates the release of dopamine and glutamate, which results in a calming effect.[14,20,21] CBD has been shown to be an agonist of 5-HT1a serotoninergic receptors and to regulate stress response as well as compulsive behaviours.[14,19,21,22]

- **Anticonvulsant effects**. The possible anticonvulsant effects of CBD are due to the inhibition of **FAAH**, the enzyme responsible for AEA degradation. Recent studies suggest CBD is targeting **FABPs** (fatty acid-binding proteins). These are intracellular proteins that mediate AEA transport to its catabolic enzyme FAAH.[16,23] By inhibiting FAAH, CBD increases levels of AEA. The anandamide function is **anticonvulsant** and **neuroprotective**.

- **Anti-nausea and antiemetic effects**. The anti-nausea and antiemetic effects of CBD may be mediated by indirect activation of somatodendritic 5-HT1A receptors.[24] **Attenuation of the mesolimbic reward system**. CBD has the ability to attenuate the mesolimbic reward system in the brain[25] and may be useful in the treatment of addictions.

- **2-AG release stimulation**. CBD stimulates the release of 2-AG.[26] This endocannabinoid plays an important role in the organism, one of them being the suppression of seizures.[27] It is also thought to play an important role in the regulation of appetite, immune system functions and pain management.

- **Antagonist at the GPR55 receptor**. CBD acts as an antagonist at the GPR55 receptor. This receptor is found in the brain, especially cerebellum, as well as in the spleen, intestine, testis, and breast tissues. It is involved in many physiological processes including bone density.[28]An overactive GPR55 receptor is associated with osteoporosis and rapid progression of various types of cancer. By working as a GPR55 antagonist, CBD may slow down the development of osteoporosis and cancer cell proliferation.[29]

- **Inhibition of the expression of ID-1 gene**. CBD inhibits the expression of ID-1 gene, which is implicated in many kinds of aggressive cancer, including brain and breast cancer.[30]

- **Agonist at PPARs**. CBD acts as an agonist at PPARs, a receptor situated on the surface of the cell's nucleus. This receptor inhibits cancer cellular growth.[31]

- **Other benefits.** CBD is also a potent anti-inflammatory, antioxidant, antipsychotic and has been shown to have neuroprotective properties.[20]

Other Cannabinoids

The two major cannabinoids in the cannabis plant are THC and CBD, apart from which it contains hundreds of other cannabinoids, or so-called minor cannabinoids.[32]

The commonly known minor cannabinoids include:

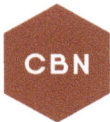

CBN

Cannabinol

CBC

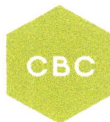

Cannabichromene

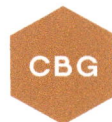

CBG

Cannabigerol

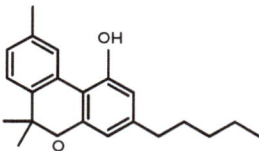

Cannabinol (CBN)

CBN is the product of THC oxidisation. It is more present in old or poorly stored cannabis. It is known to be a powerful sedative without psychoactive properties.

Other health benefits include its use as an antibacterial, anti-inflammatory, analgesic, anticonvulsant, appetite stimulant and promoter of bone cell growth. It might be useful in the treatment of burns and psoriasis.[33]

Cannabichromene (CBC)

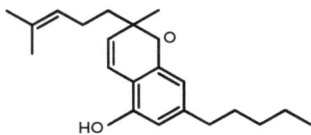

CBC is the product of enzymatic process in the plant. In this process **cannabigerolic acid (CBGA)** is converted into **cannabichromenic acid (CBCA)**. CBCA is transformed into CBC when exposed to heat (decarboxylation).

Important health benefits of CBC include its antimicrobial, anti-viral, analgesic, anti-depressant properties. It could possibly play an important role in neurogenesis and as anti-proliferative.[34]

Cannabigerol (CBG)

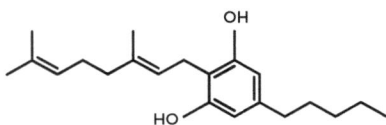

CBG is extracted from budding cannabis plants during the flowering stage. Industrial hemp contains higher levels of CBG than most cannabis strains. Breeders are now able to produce strains with a recessive gene that increases CBG levels.

CBG may have health benefits in antifungal, anti-cancer, antibacterial, neuroprotective, analgesic and antidepressant treatments. It is also potentially useful in treatment of psoriasis because of its ability to inhibit keratinocyte formation.[35]

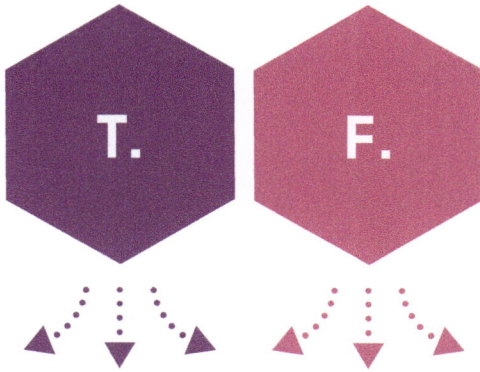

Terpenes and Flavonoids

Terpenes and **flavonoids** play a significant role in boosting the therapeutic effects of the plant, as described in the entourage effect, covered later in this section. These important compounds are synthesised in secretory cells inside the **glandular trichomes** of the cannabis plant.

The well-known terpenes include:

- **Myrcene** - Known for its sedative, analgesic and anti-inflammatory effects.[36]
- **Limonene** - One of the most abundant terpenes in cannabis. Its medicinal properties include antioxidant, anticancer, anxiolytic, antidepressant, anti-inflammatory and immune stimulation.[36]
- **Pinene** - May alleviate short-term memory impairment from THC by inhibiting acetylcholinesterase.[37]
- **Beta-caryophyllene** - Important anti-inflammatory, analgesic and selective full agonist at the CB2 receptor, it also exhibits protective properties in the stomach.[37]

Cannabis flavonoids also possess important therapeutic properties, e.g.

- **Apigenin** - Inhibits TNF-α (tumour necrosis factor), an important contributor to the development of multiple sclerosis and rheumatoid arthritis.[7]
- **Cannflavin A** - Inhibits PGE-2 (prostaglandin responsible

for inflammation) 30 times more potently than aspirin.[7]

Cannabinoid Deficiency Syndromes

Some scientists postulate that deficiencies in the endocannabinoid system may be a possible cause of many medical conditions, particularly those related to the immune system and inflammation.

In certain cases, our bodies don't produce enough endocannabinoids or enough receptors for the ECS to function properly. As a result, the body is unable to maintain homeostasis.

This theory was first put forward in 2004 by Dr Ethan Russo, who concluded in his research review that "migraine, fibromyalgia, irritable bowel syndrome and related conditions display common clinical, biochemical and pathophysiological patterns. This suggests an underlying clinical endocannabinoid deficiency that may be suitably treated with cannabinoid medicines".[38]

It may be possible that by introducing non-psychoactive cannabinoids to our body like CBD, CBDa, CBN, CBG and CBC we can potentially regulate our endocannabinoid system and prevent ECS deficiency.[39]

Endocannabinoid ciencies may implicate number of illnesses[38], Parkinson's disease, ton's disease, multiple

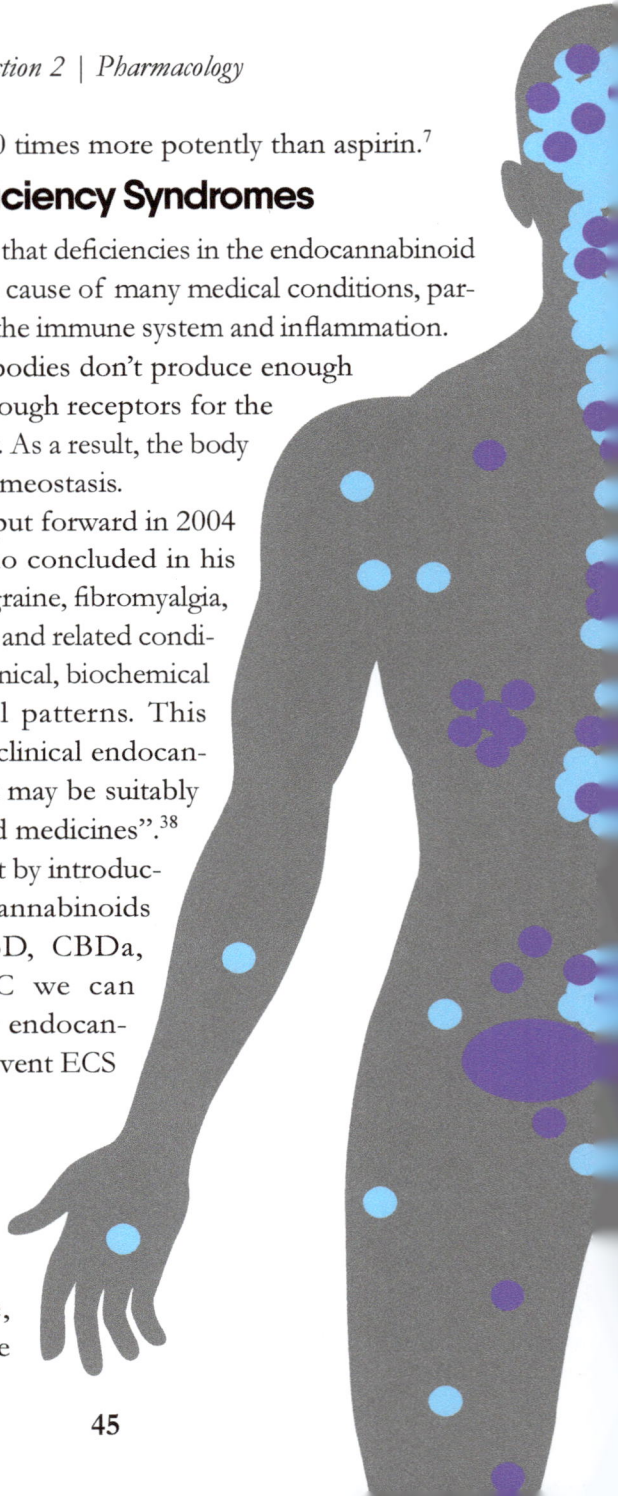

schizophrenia, fibromyalgia, anorexia nervosa, menstrual symptoms, irritable bowel syndrome, chronic motion sickness, migraine and PTSD.

There is some preliminary evidence suggesting deficiencies in the ECS are a plausible explanation of the above illnesses. However, further extensive research is required to fully understand how this may occur.

Cannabis Pharmacology

Cannabis is a versatile, multi-target therapeutic agent that has the ability to interact with the human body through the ECS[40] by activating CB1 and CB2 receptors, as well as many other metabolic pathways.[41]

THC exerts most of its actions via the endocannabinoid system.[42] CBD has a weak affinity to cannabinoid receptors and exerts its effects by interacting with other biochemical pathways in human body.[14] The minor cannabinoids, terpenes and flavonoids, are responsible for therapeutic effects as well.[43]

According to Dr Russo's cannabinoid deficiency syndrome theory, many medical conditions, especially ones related to immune system and inflammation, may be due to the deficiency in the endocannabinoid system.

It is possible that some patients are not making enough receptors or endocannabinoids for this system to work efficiently in maintaining health and homeostasis. Cannabis has the potential to balance this deficiency and provide an effective treatment option for these conditions.

In medicinal cannabis treatment, we are dealing with a whole-plant medicine and not a single- molecule synthetic agent. As per entourage effect theory, full-spectrum medicinal cannabis products provide the most synergism for desired results to take place.

Properties and actions of cannabinoids that might be of therapeutic use include:[44]

- analgesia
- muscle relaxation
- immunosuppression
- anti-inflammation
- anti-allergic effects
- sedation

- improvement of mood
- stimulation of appetite
- anti-emesis
- lowering of intraocular pressure
- bronchodilation
- neuroprotection and antineoplastic effects

Although more evidence is needed, following are some of the medical conditions that have been researched as possibly receptive to treatment with cannabis:

- Various forms of chronic pain, including migraines
- Fibromyalgia
- Chemotherapy induced nausea and vomiting
- Palliative care
- Many forms of cancer
- Epilepsy
- Pain and spasticity associated with multiple sclerosis
- Gastrointestinal problems, e.g. irritable bowel syndrome
- Neurodegenerative disease, e.g. Parkinson's disease, Alzheimer's disease, ALS
- Dystonia
- Diabetes
- Osteoporosis
- Tourette's syndrome
- Hepatitis C
- MRSA

Whole Plant Medicine & The Entourage Effect

The term "entourage effect" was coined in 1998 by Israeli scientists Shimon Ben-Shabat and Raphael Mechoulam.[45,46] It conveys the idea that each part of the plant on its own is not as effective as them all working together.[47]

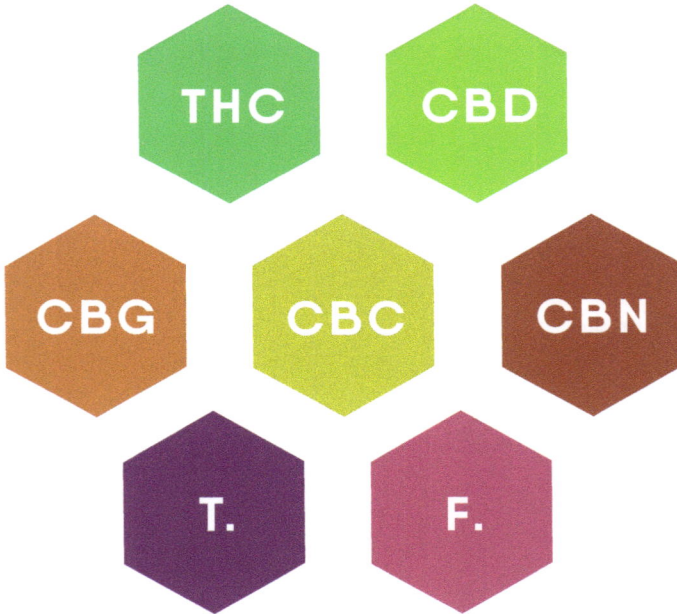

THC CBD
CBG CBC CBN
T. F.

Compounds work together, synergistically, supporting each other to produce the desired therapeutic effect

The whole-plant medicine concept became foreign to modern health professionals following the introduction of single-molecule synthetic agents. Doctors have been trained to trust these drugs as efficient, safe and predictable, in contrast to herbal medicine.

This fragmentary approach led to the extensive poly-pharmacy. Nowadays it is quite common for patients to use anything between 15-20 different drugs for different symptoms as well as using one drug to counteract the side effects of the other. Unfortunately, this leads to multiple problems, including death from overdosing.

Cannabis plant is not just THC or CBD. It contains hundreds of different cannabinoids as well as a variety of different terpenes and flavonoids, which also have their own unique therapeutic properties.[48] These compounds work together, synergistically, supporting each other to produce the desired therapeutic effect that is greater than the sum of their parts. For example, CBD modulating the psychoactive properties of THC is part of the entourage effect.[1]

In general, the whole-plant cannabis extracts are better tolerated by patients than synthetic THC and cause fewer side effects such as dysphoria, anxiety, panic reactions, paranoia and depersonalisation.[47]

The entourage effect indicates that the whole-plant medicine approach is an important part of using cannabis as a therapeutic agent.

Clinical

Applications

Chronic Pain

Chronic pain is one of the most common presentations in general practice and one of the most common reasons for patients to seek medicinal cannabis treatment.

It can be classified into three main categories:

- **Visceral** (internal organs)
- **Somatic** (skin and deep tissue)
- **Neurogenic** (nerves)

According to BUPA, about 20 per cent of adults and up to 80 per cent of Australia's nursing home residents suffer from chronic pain.[1]

It is becoming a significant public health issue, estimated to be costing the national economy more than $34 billion each year in treatment costs and lost time at work.

The most common reason, accounting for about 38 per cent of all cases, is **injury,** while about one third of chronic-pain patients are unable to identify the original cause. Other causes include arthritis, musculoskeletal conditions, headaches, cancer-related pain, post-surgical persistent pain, neuropathic pain and non-specific lower back pain.

Women tend to be more affected than men and it is usually predominant in the over-50s demographic.

Chronic pain is accompanied by **other comorbidities** including depression, anxiety, PTSD, insomnia and drug addiction.[2] It tends to affect many aspects of the patients' lives: **mental, emotional, physical, professional and social**. They are often operating in survival mode, feeling worthless and hopeless. Dealing with pain becomes a full-time job.

The usual remedy is a **cocktail of heavy medications:** opioids, benzos, antidepressants, anticonvulsants and/or NSAIDs.

These do not fully control pain and are often associated with significant adverse effects. For example, commonly used opioids, while controlling pain, may cause excessive sedation, dizziness, nausea, vomiting and/or constipation. Patients often report feeling like "zombies" and being unable to function the way they used to. Their search of pain relief often ends up in dependency and addiction.

Analgesic mechanisms of action

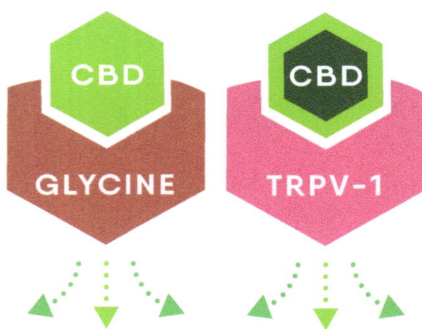

Cannabis improves pain by activating CB1 and CB2 receptors. It modulates pain perception at the level of peripheral nerves, spinal cord and brain, as well as downregulating inflammation. Studies reveal THC and CBD reduce pain associated with some forms of cancer, neuropathy and spasticity.[3,4,5]

CBD acts as an agonist to the TRPV-1 receptor. This receptor is involved in the mediation of pain perception, inflammation and body temperature.[6] It also interacts with glycine receptors which are responsible for mediation of neuropathic pain and inflammation.[6,7,8]

Cannabis can help anxiety, depression and PTSD, conditions commonly associated with chronic pain. It may improve functionality as well. Cannabis has potential to be an effective treatment option for patients suffering from chronic debilitating pain. It can be used to treat many symptoms and conditions associated with pain simultaneously, thus reducing the need for polypharmacy. In some cases, patients are able to reduce or even stop other medications.[9]

This plant has the ability to improve functionality and quality of life and in my experience its side-effects profile is superior to commonly prescribed conventional pharmaceuticals.

Here is the story shared by one of my patients:

"My life was a mess. Chronic pain had ended my career and all I loved. With the depression, chronic fatigue and other illnesses, it dragged me to the bottom of the pit. Almost bedridden, I was desperate for release from pain and a life which was bereft of joy.

With help from friends, I managed to start medical cannabis treatment in late June 2018. Progress was slow at first, but almost immediately I found my mood had improved along with a feeling of being better able to cope with my symptoms. Continuing under my doctor's expert guidance, I am now, 6 months later, feeling significant improvement in my symptoms and have removed 9 drugs (or 50%) from my daily dose of meds. That's an incredible relief for my liver which has been damaged by the use of these heavy drugs for the last 16 years.

Medical cannabis has a strangely subtle way of working on you. It does not "kick in" like opioids. It just suddenly becomes an "absence" of pain. A generalised feeling of being better in one's self. Pain which was once unbearable, becomes bearable and in some cases, non-existent. You feel better able to cope. And the great joy of it all, is that there are no crippling or biologically damaging side-effects.

Australia must make medical cannabis available to ALL who need it and most especially AFFORDABLE for all who need it. Medical cannabis has the potential to save and change lives. We must move forward with this quickly. Peoples' lives hang in the balance while we dither."

Lisa

Drug Addictions and Opioid Epidemic

In 2012, worldwide estimates on the total number of people aged 15 to 64 who used illicit substances ranged between 162 million and 324 million. Approximately 183,000 deaths were thought to be drug related.[10]

Prescription opioids are easier to obtain in the street than heroin. Predictably, deaths from prescription opioids overdose now exceed deaths attributed to heroin.

According to the Australian Bureau of Statistics, the largest proportion of deaths from prescription opioids in this country occurs within the 35-44-year-old age group (40 per cent).

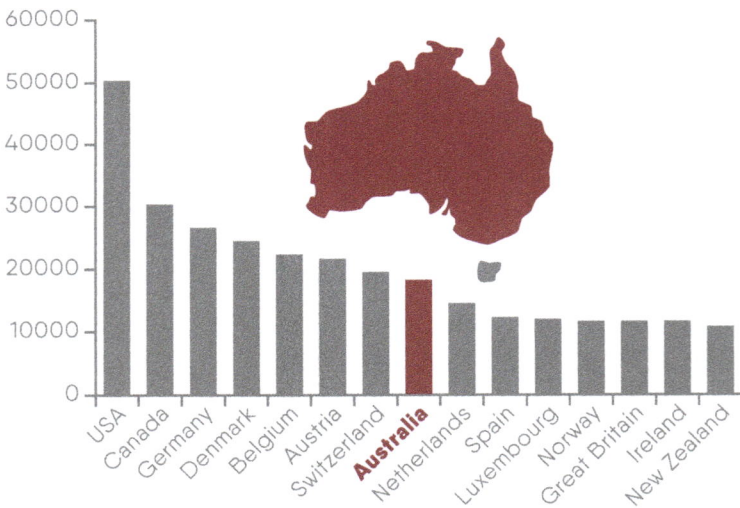

Australia ranks eighth among the world's top 30 users

Prescription drug abuse in Australia is an increasing problem. Opioid dispensing episodes have increased from 500,000 pre-scriptions in 1992 to 7.5 million prescriptions in 2012.[11] About 20,000 doses per 1 million people are prescribed daily. Further-more, data reveals that between 2009 and 2015, 80 per cent of

55

deaths from overdose were caused by pharmaceutical drugs, the most common being opioids and benzodiazepines.[11]

Australia ranks eighth among the world's top 30 users. The United States and Canada top the list.[12] Meanwhile, states in the US where cannabis has been legalised report a trend of decreasing opioid use.[13]

CBD may have therapeutic properties useful in the treatment of addiction to opioids, cocaine and psychostimulants. Some preliminary data suggests it may also be beneficial in curbing cannabis and tobacco addiction.[10]

The possible CBD mechanisms of action in the treatment of addictions:

- Acting on several neurotransmission systems involved in addiction.[14]
- Attenuating reward facilitating properties of opioids.[14]
- Anxiolytic, antipsychotic, antidepressant, along with neuroprotective properties.[15]
- Modulating psychoactive properties of THC.[16]
- Stimulating the TRVP1 receptor, thus helping body aches experienced during withdrawals.[17]
- CBD has been shown to be an agonist of 5-HT1a serotoninergic receptors, helping with depression and anxiety.[10,18]
- Regulating stress response and compulsive behaviours.[7,10]
- Allosteric modulation of opioid receptors and possible facilitation of the opioid sparing effect.[19]

CBD is shaping up as a promising therapeutic agent in the treatment of substance-use disorders. It has been associated with many neural circuits involved in the acquisition of addiction and subsequent drug-seeking behaviours. Furthermore, cannabis may play an important role in reducing opioid use due to its opioid sparing effect – an attribute I have already observed among my patients.

Cancer

Cannabis may not necessarily cure cancer but may help with symptoms associated with this disease. There are many anecdotal stories of healing cancer with cannabis. I believe that this plant shows a significant potential in this area of medicine and can be used in conjunction with conventional approaches, increasing the possibility of positive therapeutic outcomes. The ongoing and rigorous research is necessary.

Possible anti-cancer mechanisms of action include:

- **Antiproliferative** - cannabis has been found to slow down proliferation of various cancers, including breast, bladder and lung cancers.[20,21]
- **Anti-metastatic** - it may prevent cancer cells from spreading.[20,21]
- **Anti-angiogenic** - it might block the development of new blood vessels to tumour cells.[20,21]
- **Apoptosis** – may assist in programmed cell death.[20,21]
- **Inhibition of the expression of ID-1 gene** - this gene is associated with tumour growth and is implicated in several kinds of aggressive cancers including breast and brain cancers.[21]
- **Interacting antagonistically with GPR55 receptor** - this receptor, when overactive, can lead to rapid growth of several forms of cancer. By blocking signalling of this receptor cannabis may slow down cancer progression.[22]
- **Activating PPARs** - these receptors, located on the surface of the cellular nucleus, inhibit cancer growth.[23]

Cannabis might be effective in the treatment of various cancers, including:

- Brain (glioma)[24]
- Breast [24]
- Colon [24]
- Liver [24]
- Lung [20],[21]
- Prostate [24]
- Skin [25]

In summary, while more research is needed, cannabis promises to be an effective anti-cancer agent, selectively killing cancer cells while protecting the health of others.

Chemotherapy Induced Nausea and Vomiting

Chemotherapy-induced nausea and vomiting (CINV) is the most debilitating, most feared and yet most common adverse effect associated with cancer treatment. An estimated 70-80 per cent of patients undergoing chemotherapy experience CINV. This can result in significant morbidity, increased incidence of depression, anxiety and generally poor quality of life[26] as well as non-compliance leading to poor treatment outcomes.[27]

CINV is also associated with increased use of healthcare resources and economic burdens on caregivers.[27]

Conventional anti-emetics often do not fully control CINV and are associated with some adverse effects.[28]

During my own brush with breast cancer 18 years ago, anti-emetics caused severe constipation and I experienced a very unpleasant metallic taste in my mouth due to chemotherapy. For three weeks everything was completely tasteless.

The aetiology of CINV is complex and involves a network of neuroanatomical and peripheral centres, neurotransmitters and receptors.[28]

Possible cannabis anti-emetic mechanisms of action include:

- Cannabis interacts with the endocannabinoid system and many other metabolic pathways in our bodies. The ECS plays an important role in the regulation of nausea and vomiting in humans as well as animals.[29]
- Cannabis can produce an antiemetic effect by acting as **agonists to central CB1 receptors**.[30] This interaction can prevent the pro-emetic effects of endogenous compounds such as dopamine and serotonin. Worth noting is the fact that cannabinoids have been used effectively for treating CINV since 1985.[31]
- CB1 agonism suppresses vomiting and THC is the molecule acting agonistically with these receptors.[32]
- CBD suppresses nausea and vomiting as well. This effect might be mediated by interaction with 5-HT1A receptors in the brainstem.[33]
- Cannabinoids may also improve the appetite of chemotherapy patients.
- Cannabis might be useful in the treatment of chemotherapy induced neuropathy as well as helping insomnia, depression and cancer-related pain.[34]

Although more research is needed, there is a large body of anecdotal evidence supporting cannabis use in this most debilitating treatment process.

The report from the National Academies of Science Engineering and Medicine published in 2017 concluded the following:

'Furthermore, in adults with chemotherapy-induced nausea and vomiting,

there was conclusive evidence that certain oral cannabinoids were effective in preventing and treating those ailments." [35]

Palliative Care

Palliative care is a medical specialty dealing with symptom relief for patients suffering from serious, life-limiting or incurable illness. Its main focus is to provide symptoms control and improve quality of life while minimising side effects of medications. It provides holistic care addressing many aspects of serious illnesses - **physical, emotional, mental** and **spiritual**.[36]

Not all patients under palliative care suffer from terminal illness where death is expected to occur in a relatively short period of time, for example patients suffering from multiple sclerosis, heart and lung disease, neurodegenerative diseases or HIV/AIDS.[37]

Palliative care requires the use of multiple medications, some of which **control symptoms** while others **control the side effects** of these medications. Unfortunately, this approach has led to a significant polypharmacy and increased risk of serious adverse effects. For example, commonly used opioids, while controlling pain, may cause excessive sedation, dizziness, nausea, vomiting, constipation, physical dependence, tolerance, and respiratory depression.[38] For this reason, more medicines need to be used to mitigate these problems.

As a result of this multi-drug treatment many patients fall into a zombie-like state that renders them unable to function and interact with loved ones in the way they once did.[37]

Cannabis has the ability to interact with the endocannabinoid system and many other metabolic pathways in the body, thus being able to relieve so many of the patient's symptoms and to improve overall quality of life.[37,39]

It can reduce pain, help in depression, anxiety and insomnia.[40,41] In the case of terminally ill cancer patients, it may also alleviate debilitating nausea and vomiting as well as help appetite.[37] In some cases, cannabis may help to reduce or even eliminate the need to take other medications.[42]

Unfortunately, the use of cannabis in palliative care is still challenging for many health professionals following 80 years of prohibition, false dogma, prejudice and lack of understanding.

Some quote lack of evidence about its efficacy, safety and long-term side effects. It is not accurate analysis, as there is a wealth of information in thousands of reputable, scientific papers to be found online. Moreover, in the case of terminally ill patients, long-term effects are not a relevant problem.

Furthermore, doctors tend to rely heavily on the formalised evidence-based scientific research of their peers, which in the case of cannabis has been difficult because of the long-standing legality issues that surround its use.

Since March 2018, I have been able to prescribe medicinal cannabis for eight patients suffering cancer-related pain. Four of them passed away.

I have observed multiple benefits in this patient group. These include improvements in their pain, mood, appetite, overall quality of life and decreased frequency in their use of other drugs.

Following is a testimonial from the family of one of my patients:

"Alya passed away on Wednesday 3rd of October at 13:40. We are extremely grateful for your support of the past months. Without you we wouldn't have seen the extension to Alya's prognosis. I was pleased (it was wonderful but extremely hard) to have her at home a couple of times in the final weeks. Medicinal cannabis enabled the doctors to keep Alya's opioids and morphine-based medications to a minimum. Keeping these medications down gave the family time to interact with a lucid version of Alya, as prior

to the introduction of medicinal cannabis Alya was regularly detached and would retreat to the bedroom for rest/sleep. Medicinal cannabis was providing a background level of pain relief, improved her appetite and we would witness her consuming all her meals and more (as we would bring extra. She loved prawn gyoza). Medicinal cannabis helped improve her blood results and after 6 weeks on MC her bloods returned better than her entry into Royal North Shore Hospital about 3 months ago. After 7 weeks her bloods returned even better results."

In spite of the lack of proper studies, my own experiences as a GP and emerging evidence and anecdotal stories suggest that when conventional medications fail, cannabis may offer an effective and safe multi-system symptom relief for patients dealing with serious and terminal diseases.

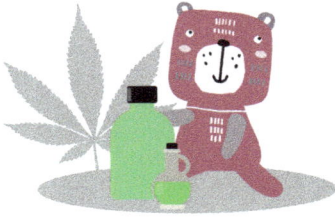

Epilepsy

The stories of children suffering from severe, intractable epilepsy (Dravet syndrome) have captured public attention over the last few years. Their suffering is immense, with some experiencing 50-100 seizures a day. Traditional pharmaceutical agents are often ineffective and present many side effects.[43]

Out of desperation and helplessness, some of the caregivers reach out for cannabis medicine. In many cases, results verge on a miracle. Documented frequencies of up to 100 seizures a day have turned into one to three a month.

Among the famous stories of children's lives being transformed is one involving a little girl named Charlotte. She was successfully treated with a formulation high in CBD, now known as Charlotte's Web.

This potential mechanism of action in epilepsy is still not fully understood. Some studies revealed that CBD may raise the threshold requirement after one action potential, making it more difficult for subsequent action potentials to fire and propagate seizure activity.[44] CBD also inhibits FAAH, the enzyme responsible for degradation of anandamide[45], the endocannabinoid which possesses neuroprotective and anticonvulsant functions.[46,47]

Furthermore, THC possesses important anticonvulsant properties and may regulate neuronal excitability.[44]

Other potential anticonvulsant mechanisms of cannabis include:

- Modulation of calcium release in neurons. Excess calcium release is neurotoxic and causes neuronal excitability.[45]
- Modulation of low-voltage-activated (T-type) Ca2+ channels, important modulators of neuronal excitability.[45]

- Reduction in glutamate toxicity, an excitatory neurotransmitter.[48]

Anecdotal evidence is significant but more research is needed to improve our understanding of the role of cannabis in the treatment of epilepsy.

Multiple Sclerosis

Multiple sclerosis (MS) can be defined as chronic, typically progressive autoimmune disease in which our body's own immune system acts against the sheaths of nerve cells (myelin) in the brain and spinal cord.

As demonstrated by the graph below MS involves many systems and causes many health issues:

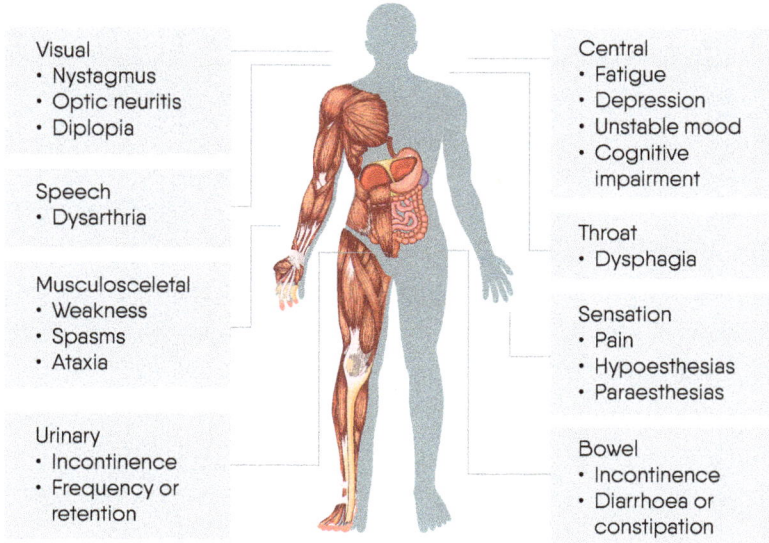

Visual
- Nystagmus
- Optic neuritis
- Diplopia

Speech
- Dysarthria

Musculosceletal
- Weakness
- Spasms
- Ataxia

Urinary
- Incontinence
- Frequency or retention

Central
- Fatigue
- Depression
- Unstable mood
- Cognitive impairment

Throat
- Dysphagia

Sensation
- Pain
- Hypoesthesias
- Paraesthesias

Bowel
- Incontinence
- Diarrhoea or constipation

Main Symptoms of Multiple Sclerosis

Spasticity is one of the major symptoms of MS. It causes overactive reflexes, involuntary movements, pain, difficulty with maintaining hygiene, abnormal posture, contractures, bone and joint deformities. MS affects every aspect of the patient's life and unfortunately there is currently no cure.

Emerging evidence supports the usage of medicinal cannabis in treating symptoms associated with MS, including:[49,50]

- Disability and disease progression
- Pain and spasticity
- Bladder function
- Ataxia and tremor
- Insomnia
- Inflammation
- Quality of life

Here is the story from one of my patients:

"My name is Christian. I'm a professional writer and in 2014, after a week in bed with my left side paralysed, I was diagnosed with Multiple Sclerosis. M.S. is mainly a disease of pain and fatigue. The nervous system attacks the brain and spinal cord, creating false and strange signals the brain doesn't deal well with. So, it causes phantom signals, a very painful case of 'pins and needles sensation'. In my case, cramps are bad enough to tear muscles. It creates 'brain fogs', where short term memories don't form easily, where cognition slows and what was a simple task yesterday becomes a fiendish puzzle the next.

To deal with this, I was prescribed Lyrica, a nerve pain agent, which was, yes, effective, but with poor psychological side effects, for me, pessimistic moods. And serious weight gain. Other medicines have had their place. I found Naprogesic useful. But not strong.

However, starting cannabis oil, a simple half-a-syringe twice a day, has been by far the most effective medication. With no real side effects, it has eased my pain, made my sleep more relaxing, lifted my mood and has certainly made sites of old cramping, often quite formidably painful, far easier to cope with. It has made my relationship with my body more positive. It's not an exaggeration to say this medicine has changed my life qualitatively for the better."

Christian

We are continuing to learn how cannabis might work in MS. According to Pertwee et al, pre-clinical evidence supports the hypothesis that activation of CB2 receptors expressed by T-cells within the central nervous system will decrease inflammation in MS.[51] This could also possibly slow down the progression of the disease.

Possible mechanisms of action might include:[52]

- Inhibition of pathogenic T-cells
- Reduction of microglial activation
- Neuroprotective, antioxidant and anti-inflammatory properties

Based on patient stories, anecdotal evidence and research, I am confident cannabis might provide multi-symptom relief for people suffering from this chronic and debilitating disease.

Neurodegenerative Diseases

Neurodegenerative diseases such as **Amyotrophic Lateral Sclerosis, Parkinson's, Alzheimer's and Huntington's** diseases occur as a result of the **neurodegenerative processes**. These processes are characterised by the progressive loss of structure and function of neurons.[52]

Cannabis can slow down the progression of neurodegenerative diseases through its **neuroprotective, antioxidant and**

anti-inflammatory properties. It has the ability to suppress excitotoxicity, glial activation and oxidative injury.[47]

It can improve **cells' mitochondrial function** and activate cellular **debris clearance**, thus improving neuron health.[53] THC has been shown to prevent **free radical damage** and encourage the **formation of new mitochondria**.[54]

Cannabinoids have been shown to reduce the effects of amyloid plaques, reduce inflammation and enhance neurogenesis in patients with Alzheimer's disease.[55] Moreover, animal studies show cannabis can reverse the ageing processes in the brain.[56]

Furthermore, cannabis can be used to treat many symptoms associated with this debilitating disease group. It can, for example, reduce tremors, rigidity and bradykinesia in Parkinson's disease.[57] It can also help with anxiety, depression, pain and behavioural problems.[56]

In summary, cannabis promises to be an effective treatment option in neurodegenerative diseases addressing many aspects of this disease group.

Diabetes

Diabetes is recognised as the world's fastest-growing chronic condition, as all countries report increasing numbers of people with type 2 diabetes. In 2013, diabetes caused 1.5 million deaths globally. Higher blood glucose levels also caused an additional 2.2 million deaths, by increasing the risks of cardiovascular and other diseases. In 2015, the 7th edition of the International Diabetes Federation's (IDF) Diabetes Atlas estimated that one in 11 adults worldwide (415 million) have diabetes.[58]

Current treatments include lifestyle modifications, diet, exercise, oral medications and insulin depending on the stage of the disease. Diabetes is a multisystem disease and cannabis is shaping up to be a potentially important therapeutic agent in addressing many aspects of this condition. It is also an important stepping stone to the discovery of novel diabetic drugs.

A large body of anecdotal evidence indicates that cannabis can stabilise sugar levels, however, scientific research to support this is still quite limited. One of the studies was published in the American Journal of Medicine in 2013. Researchers found lower levels of fasting insulin, improved insulin resistance and smaller waist size in cannabis users.[59]

Cannabis possesses potent anti-inflammatory properties. It can suppress arterial inflammation, thus reducing the incidence of cardiovascular disease. It can also improve neuropathic pain, a common diabetic complication. Some studies postulate that cannabis might improve blood pressure, thus further improving cardiovascular diabetic complications.

One of the common complications of diabetes is diabetic retinopathy, one of the leading causes of blindness in the Western world. Studies indicate that CBD, the non-psychoactive component of cannabis, might play an important role in the prevention and treatment of this important diabetic complication.[60]

In 2015 researchers at the Hebrew University of Jerusalem released a study showing that CBD could be used to treat diabetes type 2.

I believe cannabis has a strong potential in the treatment of diabetes because of its ability to address this complex, multisystem disease on multiple levels.

Inflammatory Disorders

Inflammation is the body's response to harmful stimuli such as pathogens, damaged cells or irritants. It is a protective mechanism which involves immune cells, blood vessels and molecular mediators.

The function of inflammation is to eliminate the initial cause of cell injury and to initiate tissue repair. The classical signs of inflammation are heat, pain, redness, swelling and loss of function.

Examples of disorders associated with inflammation include:
- Asthma
- Autoimmune diseases
- Autoinflammatory diseases
- Celiac disease
- Chronic prostatitis
- Colitis
- Diverticulitis
- Hay fever
- Atherosclerosis
- Rheumatoid arthritis
- Acne vulgaris

The role of cannabis in inflammatory disorders

Both CB1 and CB2 receptors have been found on immune cells. This suggests cannabinoids play a role in the regulation of the immune system.

Possible mechanisms of action include:
- **Induction of apoptosis** in activated immune cells.
- Suppression of pro-inflammatory cytokines and induction of T-regulatory cells at inflammatory sites.[61]

- THC possesses important anti-inflammatory properties, including inhibition of PEG-2 (inflammatory prostaglandin) synthesis, decreased platelet aggregation and inhibition of lipooxygenase. THC has 20 times the anti-inflammatory potency of aspirin and twice that of hydrocortisone.[62]

Conventionally used NSAIDs are associated with the increased risk of gastrointestinal track bleeding, myocardial infarction and cerebrovascular events. Cannabis is not causing these problems.[63]

Overall, it is emerging to show significant potential to be used as a novel anti-inflammatory agent, without the side effects of conventionally used anti-inflammatory drugs.

Anxiety, Depression & Schizophrenia

Cannabis is an intriguing plant. Many people around the world use it to self-medicate and report many beneficial, symptom-alleviating effects. However, as described by Julie Howard in The Pot Book, "it is a mixed bag". While it can help depression, anxiety and insomnia in some patients, it can lead to anxiety, panic attacks or even paranoia in others.

The variability of these results is likely due to the randomness of cannabis strains on the market, especially the black market. Patients obtaining drugs illegally rarely know which strains and what cannabinoid ratios they are getting. They may be buying different medicine each time they make a purchase.

Another possible explanation of inconsistent results is the **bi-directional effect** of cannabis. Due to individual genetic variabilities, people may respond differently depending on their genetic make-up.[63]

The unwanted psychoactive effects of cannabis can be

minimised when applied in a proper clinical setting, using high-quality standardised cannabis formulations of known cannabinoid, terpenes and flavonoid content and utilising the start low-go slow approach.

While THC is responsible for the psychoactive effects, the non-psychoactive, non-addictive, low-toxicity CBD exerts important anti-anxiety and anti-depressant effects by binding to serotonin receptors 5-HT1A. It also interacts with A1 and A2 receptors, leading to the downregulation of dopamine and glutamate, which in turn results in its calming effect.

CBD appears to have pharmacological properties similar to antipsychotic drugs. It promises to be a significant therapeutic agent in treatment of schizophrenia, with a much better side-effects profile than traditional antipsychotics.

The link between cannabis and schizophrenia is still debatable and unclear. Cannabis can cause short-term psychotic experiences, such as hallucinations and paranoia, even in healthy people. Heavy and/or early start of cannabis use, especially among young and susceptible individuals, may potentially lead to schizophrenia.

Interestingly, while cannabis use has increased over the last few decades, the incidence of schizophrenia remains at the same level, affecting about one per cent of the population.

Patient story

In November 2018, I prescribed pure CBD 100mg/ml for one of my patients who presented with a history of schizoaffective disorder, PTSD and insomnia. Following is his testimonial:

"I am 36 years old and have a history of mental illness, including schizoaffective disorder, PTSD and insomnia. I grew up in a very medically minded family who relied solely on medication. After many poor anti-psychotic medications, mood stabilisers and anti-depressants, I settled on a standard

anti-psychotic for over 20 years. While much of my mental Illness is genetic in nature, towards the end of 2018 I had major stressors, including the possibility of divorce, major concerns in my career and a major legal case. I decided to take a risk and try pure CBD oil. While the risk, cost and regulations were great, I realised that standard treatment, while it worked, only reduced my functioning, ability to live and had major side effects, including weight gain and poor cognition. After some months of treatment, and excellent support from my doctor, while the stressors where still present, my symptoms are little to none. In addition to this, I have lost over 10kgs in weight and quit smoking.

My asthma has improved and my cognitive ability is better. While this product is not perfect (for example it is difficult to transport, costly and takes a little time to work), both the money and administration work is worth it. I would encourage anyone who desires both symptom review and more wellness to make the sacrifices necessary and try it. If it doesn't work; so, what? You have tried. But if does work, you may just get your life back. God knows I did."

PTSD

Post-traumatic stress disorder (PTSD) can be defined as a complex medical condition which affects some individuals following traumatic life-threatening events such as accidents, assaults, natural disasters, wars etc. It results in experiences of intense fear, helplessness or horror for years after the incident.

This condition is often accompanied by obsessive compulsive disorder (OCD), depression, substance abuse and anxiety disorders such as panic attacks or social phobia. Patients suffer from insomnia, social isolation, negative flashbacks, avoidance and anxiety. They sometimes compare this experience to having a broken record inside their brain that they are unable to switch off.

The aetiology of PTSD is not fully understood. However, the possible mechanisms include:

Neurotransmitters' imbalance, including noradrenergic and serotonergic [64,65]

Dysregulation of the endocrine, cardiovascular, immune and autonomic nervous systems [66]

Dysregulation of the endocannabinoid system[67]

Role of Cannabis in PTSD

As mentioned previously, one of the functions of the ECS is the regulation of the ability to forget. Research shows PTSD is associated with lower plasma levels of anandamide[4] and impaired CB1 signalling, which in turn may result in impaired fear extinction.

Cannabis can help PTSD patients in many ways:

- It can help to treat various addictions, commonly associated with PTSD.[68,69]
- Medicinal cannabis can help reduce aggressive behaviours, anger and irritability, which is also common in PTSD patients.[70]
- It can improve depression, anxiety, sleep and nightmares.[71]

Many of my patients who approach me to prescribe medicinal cannabis for chronic pain also suffer from PTSD. It appears that balanced cannabis formulations, with equal THC and CBD, work quite well for many of them. Here is the story of one:

"I am 47 years old and I have PTSD (severe), chronic pain (debilitating), OCD and a number of related or associated conditions. I have an autoimmune disease and a long medical history.

Over the many decades, I have been put on every medication to treat these conditions. The lowest point was where I was told by hospitals not to bother going back (private and public) as there was nothing else they could do for me. I was taking opioids and taking different medications for many conditions - at one point there were 18 tablets per day. It got to the point that there was no option left. I had tried everything else. I was ready to die. I was comfortable with that; I knew I had tried everything that I could. In that time, I had been following the treatment of my conditions with cannabis and saw positive results. That was something I had not tried so I needed to at least try, I owed that to my son at least.

The results were dramatic. I am able to do things that people take for granted like going to a market, be in a public, go to the shops. I never thought I would be able to exercise again. I am back exercising. I describe it as chains breaking free and it has opened up a whole new life. It has stabilised my moods. I am able to control my triggers, not the triggers controlling me. Cannabis oil has put things back where they should be, exactly what medication is supposed to do.

Cannabis has saved my life and a big thank you needs to go to the Chief Medical Officer at MediHuanna for listening, for acting and just knowing I was at that point."

Damien

PTSD is a very complex clinical condition and medicinal cannabis appears to have properties alleviating many symptoms associated with this disorder. This especially holds true when used in a proper clinical setting, combined with other modalities of healing, including psychological treatments and lifestyle advice.

Osteoporosis

Osteoporosis is a medical condition in which bones become thin, weak and fragile, thus making them susceptible to fracture (break) due to minimal trauma. This disease is now considered a serious public health problem worldwide, affecting more than

200 million people, with its incidence on the rise.[71]

Approximately 30 per cent of all postmenopausal women in the United States and in Europe suffer from osteoporosis.[72] In Australia, according to Australian Health Survey, in 2011-12 self -reported diagnosed osteoporosis affected 15 per cent of women and three per cent of men over 50.[72]

Osteoporosis can be preventable and lifestyle factors play an important role. These include:

- Well-balanced diet, including calcium-rich foods
- Regular exercise
- Minimising alcohol, coffee consumption and avoiding smoking
- Current medical treatments including:
- Fosamax
- Actonel
- Prolia

Cannabis may play a significant role in the treatment of osteoporosis. Studies indicate the **endocannabinoid system** plays an important role in the regulation of bone mass in both health and disease.[73] Cannabinoid receptors CB1 and CB2 are present in the bones.

Sympathetic Nervous System is crucial in maintaining bone homeostasis[74] **CB1 receptors** are present in skeletal sympathetic nerve terminals and regulate the adrenergic tonic restrain of bone formation.[75]

CB2 receptors are expressed in osteoblasts and osteoclasts. This stimulates bone formation, and inhibits bone resorption.[76]

One of the main physiological function of CB2 receptors in the bone is maintaining bone remodelling, thus protecting the skeleton against age-related bone loss.[76]

In humans, polymorphisms in CNR2, the gene encoding CB2,

are strongly associated with postmenopausal osteoporosis.[76]

Moreover, CBD interacts antagonistically with GPR55 receptor. This receptor, when overactive, is associated with osteoporosis.[76]

To conclude, cannabis may provide another treatment option in the prevention and treatment of osteoporosis, especially when combined with the important lifestyle measures such as exercise and healthy diet.

Antibacterial & Antioxidant

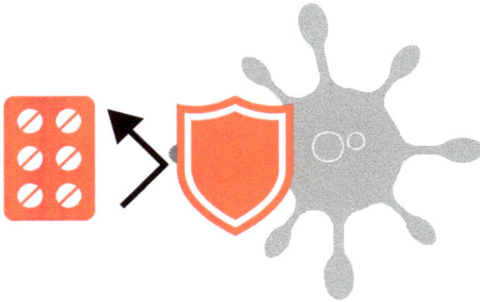

Owing to inappropriate and overuse of antibiotics, antimicrobial resistance is becoming an urgent global health priority. Its prevalence is increasing in Australia and worldwide, with common and treatable infections becoming life threatening.[77]

Unfortunately, the pharmaceutical industry is unable to keep up with the need to develop new antibiotics, while antimicrobial resistance is on the increase.[78]

Cannabis was used throughout centuries as a topical antibiotic in skin infections, erysipelas and tuberculosis.[78] Studies indicate the active compound of cannabis possesses potent antimicrobial properties.[79] All major cannabinoids have been shown to be very effective against a variety of methicillin-resistant staphylococcus aureus (MRSA).[80] This has important clinical implications as MRSA is on the increase.

Moreover, cannabis is considered one of the most potent antioxidants, with studies indicating that CBD and THC are more efficacious than both alpha-tocopherol and ascorbate.[80]

We are now facing the increased problems presented by this antimicrobial resistance and the concomitant danger of untreatable infections. Cannabis, with its antibacterial and anti-oxidative properties, might be an important therapeutic option in the treatment of various infections.

Safety Considerations

Acute Toxicity and Safety Ratio of Cannabis

Cannabis appears to be one of the safest known therapeutic agents as there are no reported deaths from overdose. However, higher amounts may increase the possibility of adverse events, especially when used concurrently with other medications.

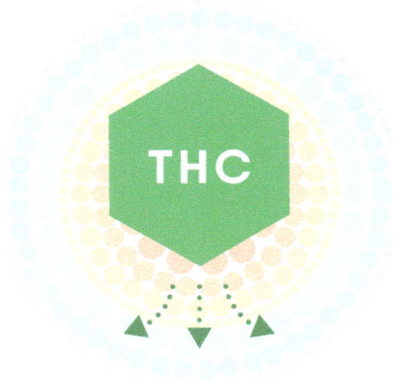

THC

>800 MG/KG
MEDIAN LETHAL DOSE OF THC:

30 MG
MAXIMUM DAILY
DOSE OF THC

Side effects are mostly related to THC, the psychoactive component of the plant, and the median lethal dose is estimated to be >800mg/kg.

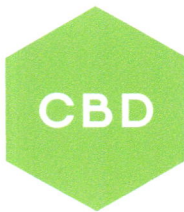

CBD

1000 MG/KG
CBD DOSE SAFELY TOLERATED

As stated previously, CBD is considered to be of very low toxicity and doses of 1000mg/kg CBD appear to be safely tolerated in humans.[1]

Cannabis has a superior safety profile in comparison to many other traditional medications.[2] While it may present a variety of side effects, many of them can be mitigated effectively in a

79

proper clinical setting.

Robert Gable conducted a study that compared a range of psychoactive substances by measuring the lethal dose and safety ratio. The results measured the usual effective dose of pure THC at 15mg, with a lethal dose being 15g. Therefore, 1,000 consecutive doses would be required to reach a lethal dose, putting the safety ratio at 1:>1000.[3]

Codeine is one of the most common pharmaceutical agents used in the treatment of chronic pain. With a usual dose measured at 40mg and a lethal dose measured at 800mg, 20 consecutive doses would represent a lethal dose, putting the safety ratio at 1:20.[3]

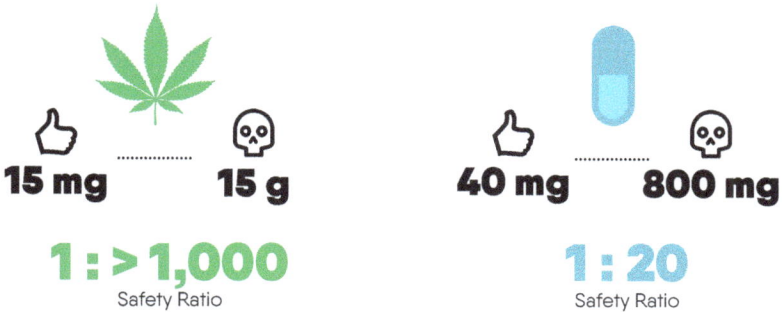

15 mg .... **15 g**

1 : > 1,000
Safety Ratio

40 mg .... **800 mg**

1 : 20
Safety Ratio

The ratios speak volumes in favour of cannabis.

Acute Lethal Toxicity – Psychoactive Substances

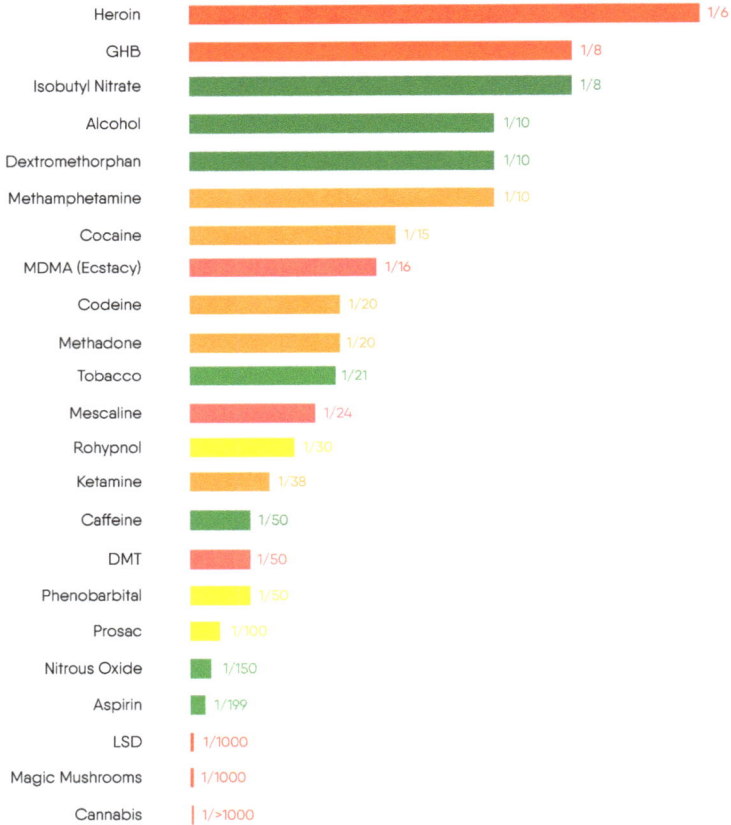

Substance	Ratio
Heroin	1/6
GHB	1/8
Isobutyl Nitrate	1/8
Alcohol	1/10
Dextromethorphan	1/10
Methamphetamine	1/10
Cocaine	1/15
MDMA (Ecstacy)	1/16
Codeine	1/20
Methadone	1/20
Tobacco	1/21
Mescaline	1/24
Rohypnol	1/30
Ketamine	1/38
Caffeine	1/50
DMT	1/50
Phenobarbital	1/80
Prosac	1/100
Nitrous Oxide	1/150
Aspirin	1/199
LSD	1/1000
Magic Mushrooms	1/1000
Cannabis	1/>1000

DEA Drug Schedules

Unscheduled – Legal over the counter

Schedule 4 or 5 – Prescribable (Low Danger)

Schedule 2 or 3 – Prescribable (Dangerous)

Schedule 1 – Illegal and Dangerous

Above graph data from Gable RS [4]

81

Physical Dependence

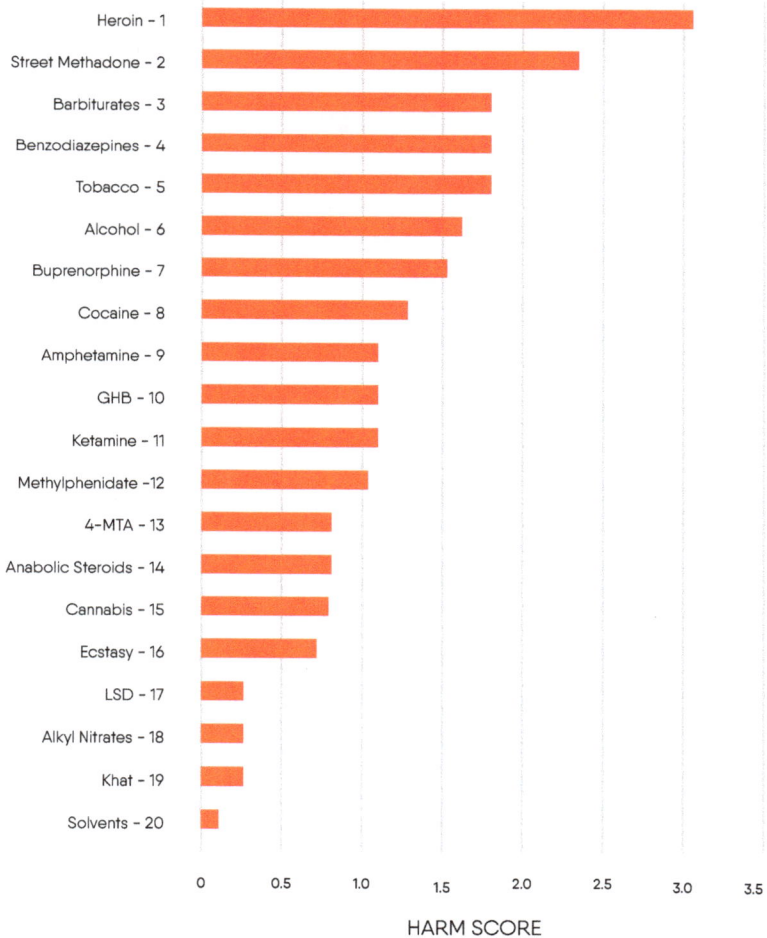

Drug	Harm Score
Heroin – 1	
Street Methadone – 2	
Barbiturates – 3	
Benzodiazepines – 4	
Tobacco – 5	
Alcohol – 6	
Buprenorphine – 7	
Cocaine – 8	
Amphetamine – 9	
GHB – 10	
Ketamine – 11	
Methylphenidate –12	
4–MTA – 13	
Anabolic Steroids – 14	
Cannabis – 15	
Ecstasy – 16	
LSD – 17	
Alkyl Nitrates – 18	
Khat – 19	
Solvents – 20	

HARM SCORE

Above graph data from Independent Scientific Committee on Drugs [5]

Critics of cannabis claim it's addictive. The reality is that cannabis has low dependence potential. It is much less addictive than alcohol, tobacco and many legally prescribed drugs, with the addiction score at around 0.8 in comparison to heroin, which scores 3.

Drug Induced & Causes of Death in Australia 2012

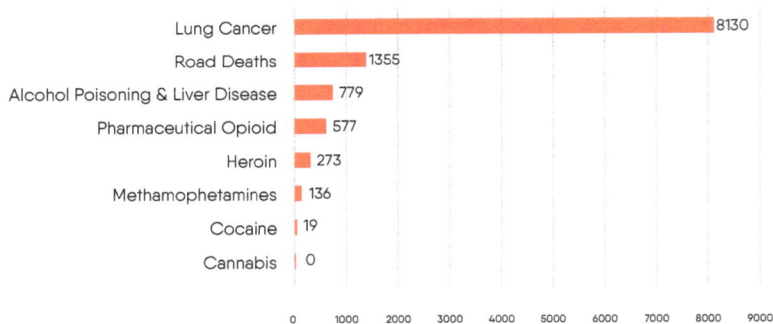

Above graph data from ABS [6] and NDARC [7,8]

As already stated, there are no reported deaths due to cannabis overdose. Interestingly, the following graph shows deaths resulting from accidental opioids overdose rank at 4 and exceed those from heroin overdose.

Short-term and Long-term effects of cannabis

Short-term effects of cannabis might include:
- Altered visual and auditory perception [9]
- High doses of THC may increase anxiety, depression,

paranoia and psychotic symptoms[9]
- Increased phlegm, cough, wheezing, and shortness of breath[9]
- Impaired short-term memory[4]
- Altered thinking[4]
- Loss of inhibition [9]
- Spontaneous laughter[7]
- Quiet and reflective mood[7]
- Confusion[7]
- Reddened/bloodshot eyes[7]
- Sleepiness[7]
- Reduced coordination and balance[7]
- Increased heart rate[7]
- Low blood pressure[7]
- Increased appetite[7]

Long-term cannabis use might cause:
- Impaired concentration, memory and learning ability[9]
- Sore throat, bronchial irritation[6]
- Changes in hormonal balance leading to lowered sex drive, irregular menstrual cycles and lowered sperm counts[10]
- Heavy and regular cannabis use may be associated with the development of "drug-induced psychosis", especially in young or susceptible individuals, however it is debatable and association is not necessarily a causation
- Smoking cannabis during adolescence might have a detrimental effect on the developing brain, lowering IQ, memory and cognition[8]
- Cannabinoid hyperemesis syndrome, possibly associated with chronic cannabis use and characterised by episodes of nausea, vomiting, thirst and frequent bathing.[11]

Potential Drug Interactions

The exogenous cannabinoids in the cannabis plant can be used to treat a variety of medical conditions. However, before commencing the treatment, it is important to understand any potential drug interactions involving these pharmacologically diverse molecules. This holds especially true when co-administering cannabis with other medications.[1]

Drug interactions with cannabis are mainly associated with simultaneous use of other CNS depressants. Clear evidence demonstrates that alcohol may increase THC levels.[12,13] Moreover, cannabis has **additive CNS depressant effects** with alcohol, barbiturates and benzodiazepines. Furthermore, THC and CBD may increase the anticoagulant effect of warfarin, hence regular INR monitoring is very important.[14]

Cannabis is metabolised in the liver, using cytochrome P450 enzymes.[1] These enzymes are responsible for the metabolism of most medications that enter the human body.

Drugs involved can act as enzyme **substrates, inducers** or **inhibitors** of **CYP450 enzymes**.[15]

- **Substrates** are molecules that are metabolised by these enzymes.
- **Inhibitors** are the molecules that reduce the activity of the enzyme, slowing the metabolism of its substrates and increasing the substrate concentration and effect.
- **Inducers** increase the activity of the enzyme, enhancing the metabolism of its substrates and decreasing the substrate concentration and effect.

Enzymes that are known to affect cannabis use include: CYP1A2, CYP3A4, CYP2C19, CYP2C9[19,2] and CYP2D6.[18]

The following enzymes may be potential contributors to the

primary metabolism of the following exogenous cannabinoids:[19]

- THC – Tetrahydrocannabinol (CYP2C9, CYP3A4)
- CBD – Cannabidiol (CYP2C19, CYP3A4)
- CBN – Cannabinol (CYP2C9, CYP3A4)

The CYP3A4, CYP2C9 and CYP2C19 enzyme is involved in the metabolism of both THC and CBD.[16] Therefore, inhibitors of these enzymes may increase the concentrations of cannabinoids, while inducers may decrease the concentrations of these cannabinoids.

THC is a CYP1A2 inducer. Theoretically, THC may decrease the concentrations of clozapine, duloxetine, naproxen, cyclobenzaprine, olanzapine, haloperidol, and chlorpromazine. Smoking cannabis may also cause induction of the CYP1A2 enzyme,[19] which may decrease the concentrations of CYP1A2 substrates.

Additionally, CBD is a potent inhibitor of CYP2D6[18] and CYP3A4[20] and may increase serum concentrations of drugs metabolised by the CYP2D6 and CYP3A4 enzyme.

It is interesting that CBD may have significant effects in the treatment of epilepsy and has important drug interactions with anti-seizure medication. CBD may increase clobazam levels, a very important consideration in the treatment of refractory epilepsy for children.[17]

In conclusion, most potential interactions with cannabinoids through the inhibition and induction of major human CYP450 isoforms are generally low risk,[14] and significant drug interactions rarely occur. If necessary, cannabis may be used in combination with other drugs.[2]

Contraindications and Precautions

- Cannabis is contraindicated in pregnant and lactating women.
- It is recommended not to use cannabis in patients with a history of psychosis except when CBD predominant formulations are used.
- Caution should be exercised when cannabis is used in unstable cardiac conditions such as angina due to tachycardia and possible hypotension caused by THC.
- While use in children and adolescence is debatable, it also depends on the medical condition being treated and when benefits clearly outweigh the risk, e.g. in intractable childhood epilepsy.
- Addiction and dependency are another debatable area, however, high CBD formulations can be useful in the treatment of drug abuse.
- Smoking is generally not recommended, in particular in patients who suffer from COPD and asthma.[2]

Patient Care

Determining Suitability for Cannabis Treatment

When considering cannabis for your patients, it essential to properly assess the suitability of that treatment for each patient on a case by case basis. During the **initial assessment** we need to discuss the patient's **expectations** because sometimes those might be quite unrealistic. As doctors, we should be upfront and honest about what we may or may not accomplish. Patients need to be made aware it may take time to get the dosing right to achieve the desired therapeutic outcome and that sometimes, products may need to be changed.

Cannabis medicine requires time and patience from both the treating physician and patient.

Affordability of cannabis is another issue that needs to be raised because it is still very expensive in Australia. The goals of treatment need to be formulated and explained to patients. These will include symptoms control, improving quality of life and reducing side effects caused by polypharmacy.[1]

As with any treatment it is important to conduct a **risk to benefit analysis** as to whether the possible benefits outweigh the potential risks. In particular, both the possible **therapeutic and adverse effects** need to be gone through. For example, caution needs to be exercised in patients who present with a history of psychotic episodes.

Currently, cannabis treatment in Australia is not a first line option. It may be used if patients aren't responding to conventional medicines or are unable to tolerate these treatments due to adverse side effects. Previous treatment history and the types of medicines trialled need to be documented, along with adverse effects experienced.

Cannabis is a versatile medicine useful in the treatment of

many complex and rare conditions where patients do not respond well to conventional treatments. At this stage in Australia, cannabis can be used in the treatment of the following conditions: epilepsy, spasticity in multiple sclerosis, chemotherapy-induced nausea and vomiting, pain and palliation.[2]

Treatment Considerations

Cannabis is a **multi-target drug**, meaning it can be used to treat multiple symptoms and conditions simultaneously. This can help to minimise the number of therapeutic agents used and reduce the need for polypharmacy.[1] Due to the entourage effect, cannabis appears to work best as a whole plant medicine.[3]

The overall therapeutic approach needs to be patient cantered and based on individual dosing using the "**start low, go slow approach**".[4]

To maintain continuity and quality of care, it is important to have **reliable access** to high quality, organic cannabis preparations with consistent cannabinoid profiles.

Medicinal cannabis products need to be extracted and processed under Good Manufacturing Practice (GMP) guidelines ensuring that all products are free of pesticides as well as microbial and heavy-metal contamination. Cannabinoid profiles of batches should also be independently tested with the verified cannabinoid ratios clearly labelled on the final product.

Biphasic Effect

The biphasic effect of cannabis means that low and high dosage can produce the opposite effects, for example small doses may have a stimulating effect while high ones may have a sedating effect. It is an important consideration when dosing.

This effect of cannabis can be utilised in the treatment of a large variety of clinical conditions. For example, in cases of insomnia and depression, higher doses can be used at night to help sleep and lower doses taken in the morning to elevate mood. It is important to keep in mind that too much THC, while not lethal, can worsen anxiety and mood disorders.[5]

CBD appears to be well tolerated at any dose. However, possible drug interactions need to be observed. Also, we need to keep in mind that less is more in respect to cannabis. Too much CBD could be less effective therapeutically than a moderate dose.

Bi-directional effect of cannabis

Cannabis is known for its bi-directional effects. It can alleviate anxiety and depression in some individuals and aggravate it in others.[6] Research indicates that these opposite effects might be due to individual genetic variabilities.[7]

Balanced Cannabinoid Ratios

Clinical experience shows that combined THC and CBD formulations are generally more effective than CBD or THC alone, especially in the treatment of pain, spasticity and insomnia.[8] Patients suffering from these conditions often require preparations higher in THC.

In contrast to the recreational users, the majority of medicinal cannabis patients often seek CBD-rich formulation with the smallest amount of THC. This approach is used to achieve the greatest improvement in symptom control, function and quality of life, with minimal adverse events.[1]

CBD dominant products have fewer untoward psychotropic effects but may require higher dosing. Moreover, CBD is known to modulate the euphoric effects of THC, which is an important consideration for daytime use.[1] For example, CBD predominant formulations may be used in the morning and products with a higher THC amount at night.

The right cannabinoid ratios are established for each individual patient based on the "start low, go slow approach". Sometimes, we start with low THC and high CBD formulations to find out in the process whether we may move to equal THC and CBD products or perhaps to those with higher THC content. This decision is based on individual patient response.

The prescribing of cannabis medicine requires a distinctly personalised approach and the concept of "one size fits all" is not going to work very well here.

Pharmacokinetic Considerations

The **onset** and **duration of action** for each cannabis dose can vary depending on how the medicine is absorbed, distributed and metabolised in the body.

Absorption has the most variability and factors such as product bioavailability, the level of fat solubility as well as organ tissue differences (lungs, skin, stomach) all play an important role. Furthermore, cannabis is a fat soluble and has a low water solubility.

For topical and oral routes, cannabis is best absorbed in the **presence of fat**. Meal timing needs to be taken into consideration when assessing dosage as this may affect **bioavailability**.

For inhalation methods, the depth of inhalation, duration of breath holding and temperature of vaporizer all affect cannabis absorption.[1]

Chemovar Considerations

There are thousands of cannabis plant breeds, commonly known as 'strains', with the preferred terms being 'chemical variety' or **'chemovar'**. Understanding the importance of chemovar variability is essential to maximising therapeutic benefits.

The numerous cannabis chemovars contain varying cannabinoid ratios and other components such as terpenes and flavonoids, with each one of these compounds having key pharmacological and modulatory effects. The varying proportions of these components determine the therapeutic and adverse effects associated with each chemovar.

In general, the majority of medicinal cannabis products are low THC and high CBD. There appears to be a misconception among some patients that they need to feel 'high' to achieve symptom control. Triggering euphoric effects of THC is generally not needed to achieve therapeutic effects.[1]

Chemovars with a combination of different cannabinoids offer broader mechanisms of action and improved therapeutic outcomes.[1]

Currently, the main types of chemovars can be classified into three categories:[1]

- Type 1: THC predominant
- Type 2: Mixed THC, CBD
- Type 3: CBD predominant

Patient Centred Considerations

Cannabis medicine needs to be patient centred and based on individual dosing because of the differences in the endocannabinoid tone among patients.[1] For this reason, it is essential to understand the complex interactions within the endocannabinoid system.

Additionally, it is important to consider the patient's **past cannabis use experience** and **addiction potential**. Patients previously exposed to cannabis may need higher doses than cannabis naive patients. The TGA suggests that cannabis-naive patients may only need 10% – 50% of the starting dose of a regular cannabis user to note effects (both positive and negative).[4]

Common side effects, especially the **psychoactive properties of THC,** also need to be addressed and mitigated against. Ideally, THC predominant formulations should be administered at bedtime to limit adverse effects and encourage tolerance development. However, this is not essential.

When treating with cannabis it is vital to consider the **different rates of metabolism** for each patient, due to the genetic variability in the hepatic metabolic pathways (slow and fast metabolisers). This is an important consideration when treating patients through the oral route because cannabis is metabolised in the liver.[9,10]

It is also important to address possible **drug interactions.** Cannabis is metabolised by **cytochrome P450,**[11] the metabolic pathway shared by many medications, so doses will need to be adjusted accordingly. Please refer to the chapter on drug interactions.

The **bidirectional effects** of cannabis need to be considered as well because, due to genetic variability, they may cause opposite outcomes, for example aggravating anxiety in some and alleviating it in others.[6] Additionally, different doses may be required for **symptom control** vs **disease modification.**[1]

Dosing & Titration

Cannabis is considered to have a superior safety profile, however several factors must be taken into account with regards to dosing and titration. Generally, the recommended approach is "start low and go slow".[1] It is important to establish the minimum effective dose so that adverse effects may be minimised and therapeutic responses optimised. Clinical observations show that patients tolerate cannabis well without significant side effects when dosing slowly and carefully.

Another important consideration is the cost to the patient, as a monthly supply of cannabis in Australia at present costs anywhere between $AUD 200-$500. Optimising the cost for the patients is another reason for finding the minimal, clinically effective dose.

Like all medicines, cannabis may have some side effects. However, these are mostly related to THC, the psychoactive component of the plant, and therefore dosing is determined by the amount of THC in each product. THC-related side effects such as fatigue, tachycardia and dizziness can be minimised when the starting dose is low and following titration is slow. Gentle increases in dose promote tolerance to the psychoactive effects of THC, which is especially important for naive users.[1]

High THC formulations may allow for the use of lower amounts but it is important that patients titrate accordingly to avoid adverse effects. It is recommended that the **maximum daily dose of THC** should not exceed **30 mg/day** unless clin-ically justified, with the benefits outweighing the possible risks.

Without improved efficacy, doses exceeding the recommended 30mg/day may increase adverse effects.[1] When considering a higher amount of THC, it is important to remember that the median lethal dose is estimated to be >800mg/kg.[4] Moreover, it is recommended to use THC in conjunction with CBD to avoid 95 psychoactive effects.[1]

Because CBD has very low toxicity and is less potent than THC, higher volumes might be required to achieve optimal results. Quantities of 1000 mg/kg CBD appear to have been safely tolerated in humans.[4] Doses of 2500 mg per day may be required in the treatment of intractable epilepsy.

The **initial daily dose of THC is 2.5 mg daily or 1.25 mg** for elderly and cannabis naive patients and increased by 2.5mg or 1.25 mg every 4-5 days until optimum results are achieved or adverse effects develop.[1] If the latter occurs, the dose should be dropped to a previously tolerated dose. It is preferred to start administering cannabis at night, especially in the case of high THC formulations. However, this is not essential.[1]

In case of Nabiximol, an oromucosal spray with a 1:1 ratio of THC and CBD, most patients require 6–8 sprays per day for symptomatic relief with a maximum dose of twelve. Higher doses may increase adverse events without improved efficacy.[1]

Patients using inhalation methods should start with one inhalation and wait 15 minutes. After that they may increase to one inhalation every 15–30 minutes until desired symptom control has been achieved.[1]

Above all else, it is important to remember that the **"start low, go slow"** approach is essential and it is generally recommended that titration should take place over a period of about two weeks.

Delivery Methods

Delivery methods

There are several ways to administer medicinal cannabis. The choice will depend on the patient's preferences, familiarity, age, medical condition and required onset and duration of action.

Common delivery methods include:

- Inhalation
- Oral
- Topical
- Rectal
- Vaginal
- Juicing

Currently in Australia, cannabis oils delivered orally are the most common mode of administration. As a clinician I'd like to see many forms of delivery widely available so they may be used according to patient needs. For example, having an option of using oral or rectal formulations on a regular basis and inhalation or sublingual ones for breakthrough symptoms e.g. pain, nausea, vomiting.

Inhalation Methods

Inhalation methods include smoking and vaping. Metered dose devices are becoming available as well.

Smoking seems to be most popular and generally preferred by patients in many parts of the world. It is not encouraged because of the toxic by-products, such as PAH (polycyclic aromatic hydrocarbons), carbon monoxide (CO) and ammonia (NH3) created through the combustion of smoke at 600-900°C.[1] Moreover, 30-50 per cent of cannabis is incinerated through this process, making it a less efficient method of delivery.[1,2] Regular smoking is often associated with respiratory symptoms such as bronchitis, cough, wheezing and increased phlegm.[1] However, studies so far don't indicate increased risk of developing COPD or lung cancer unless cannabis is mixed with the tobacco.[1]

In comparison to smoking, vaping offers a more efficient cannabinoid extraction. This process heats cannabis at 160-230°C. Toxic elements are significantly reduced but not completely eliminated.[1] Additionally, patients report less respiratory symptoms.[1]

Both methods offer quick onset of action within minutes, with the peak effect within 30 minutes and duration of action between two to four hours.[1] Bioavailability varies between 2-56 per cent.[3]

The advantage of inhalation methods is rapid onset of action, which is important for quick relief of acute symptoms, for example severe pain or nausea in terminally ill cancer patients.

As a clinician, I would like to see the metered dose devices, similar to asthma puffers, widely available. These devices would be more acceptable for many patients and allow precise dosing.

A promising product made in Israel, the Syqe Inhaler™, may do just this [4]. As part of their proprietary system, raw cannabis material is packaged into cartridges that can be inserted into the pocket-sized device and deliver a metered dose for the patient every time. The maker claims, this promises to increase dosing precision and efficiency while easing the dosing burden on patients. The analytical data captured from the device would also help treating clinicians better observe patient responses adding to quality of care.

Oral Methods

Oral cannabis products include oils, tinctures, extracts, capsules, brownies, chocolate bars, drinks, cookies, pills and snacks.

In Australian clinical situations, the most common delivery method continues to be cannabis oils taken orally. Oral cannabis preparations usually work within 30-90 minutes, with peak effects between 2-4 hours, the total duration of action usually lasting between 4-12 hours and in some cases as long as 24 hours. Bioavailability from oral based cannabis products range from 10-20 per cent.[5]

Sublingual delivery methods provide rapid effects similar to smoking without exposing the lungs to heat, tar or other unwanted collateral effects, including unpleasant smoke smell, smoky taste, dry mouth and throat irritation.[6,7]

Common examples of this type of medication include dissolvable strips, sublingual sprays and medicated lozenges.

Topical Methods

Cannabinoids can be absorbed through the skin and might be useful to alleviate localised symptoms. Examples of topical products include:

- Creams
- Balms
- Patches

The onset of action is within one to two hours and the duration of these effects is approximately six to eight hours.[7] Using ingredients to mildly disrupt skin barrier may allow better absorption of the formulation.[1]

A transdermal patch delivers cannabinoids at a controlled release rate;[8] however, this form is not widely available despite being around since 1979.[7]

Patients who have used patches report onset of action within two hours and duration of effect lasting upwards of two days.[7]

Rectal Methods

Suppositories are suitable for patients who are unable or unwilling to ingest or inhale cannabis.[9] This group includes:

- Patients suffering from chemotherapy-induced nausea and vomiting.[9]
- Elderly patients and children.[9]
- Surgical patients who are unable to eat immediately before and after operations.[9]
- Patients who are unable to swallow due to stroke or another disease. Additionally, suppositories might be effective in alleviating symptoms associated with Crohn's disease and ulcerative colitis.[9]
- Many male patients who report that suppositories are effective in treating various health problems associated with prostate.[9]

The rectal form of administration is characterised by relatively fast onset of action – 10 to 15 minutes. Duration is from four to eight hours and bioavailability 50–70 per cent.[9,10]

More scientific research is needed for this method of cannabinoid application.

Vaginal method

Vaginal delivery method was used throughout the ages, for example ancient Egyptians would grind cannabis into honey and apply the mixture to the vagina to induce contractions during labour.[11] Today, many conventional pharmaceuticals are administered through the vagina. Cannabis shouldn't be an exception here. I was unable to find a lot of information about vaginal cannabis administration. I decided to include it in this book as I believe that many women may find this cannabis application useful in treating pelvic-related problems, especially painful periods and endometriosis. This method of delivery may reduce the rate of systemic effects and produce the therapeutic outcomes where it is required. However, more research is needed.

I am aware cannabis tampons have become available in the US but I know many women don't like them. In my opinion, vaginal pessaries, creams and gels delivering various cannabis formulations would be more appropriate.

Cannabis Juicing

There is growing interest in the medicinal properties of raw cannabis. A number of patients are now juicing many parts of this plant and report multiple therapeutic benefits. This method was first popularised by Dr William Courtney.[12]

Cannabinoids in the raw plant occur in the neutral, acid form and require the process of decarboxylation through heating to become psychoactive. THCA (the acid form of THC) possesses important anti-inflammatory, anti-emetic, neuroprotective and anticonvulsant properties. CBDA (the acid form of CBD) shows potent anti-anxiety and anti-emetic properties in rodents.[1]

One of the powerful Australian medical stories is that of Morgan Taylor, who has been using cannabis juice to help with her Crohn's disease. Below is her testimonial:

"To anyone who still disputes the healing abilities of cannabis, is this enough proof? I have lived for years with excruciating pain, incontinence, malnutrition, infection, blood loss and more. Prescription drugs have left me with horrific side effects such as crippling lupus, anaphylaxis, hair loss, osteoporosis and joint pain so severe it required morphine injections and made me contemplate suicide.

Six weeks ago, I was in hospital facing the removal of my colon, rectum and abdominal muscle. Now I am healthier and happier than I have been in YEARS. I feel like I have my life back again. Raw cannabis juice has saved my life. I can say that with 100% certainty. It wasn't too long ago that I felt like giving up, but there is always hope."

Conclusion

Following a near century long failed war on cannabis it is now re-appearing in the modern world with the same purpose as its origins in ancient history. Its medicinal properties can no longer be denied, it's time to stop fighting it and instead embrace the potential it holds to heal.

Unfortunately, much misinformation and baseless propaganda still exist and it is for this reason I wrote this book, with the goal to share the truth about this plant and its therapeutic properties. It's time for us doctors to look past the propaganda fed to us throughout prohibition and take an unbiased look into cannabis as a modern medicine.

As doctors we have been trained to rely solely on evidence-based scientific research with little regard to the mystery of healing itself, the transcendental part that will never be proven in a lab or RCT. Lab studies produce the map but not the territory - and we shouldn't confuse the two. Most importantly it is time to listen with compassion to our patients and their stories of healing and hope.

I believe in balance: the continuation of rigorous scientific research while at the same time embracing the other aspects of healing. Therefore, I very much support n=1 studies, where each individual is followed as a subject of research. Combining the studies of science and metaphysics will not only improve our understanding of cannabis but other plants and synthetic therapeutic agents as well.

For too long we have missed out on the therapeutic value of cannabis due to fear tactics, however, times are changing and more research is being conducted now than ever before. This has led to an increasing number of countries moving to legalise cannabis for medicinal, acknowledging the mistakes of the past.

Conclusion

It is an exciting time in human history as we bear witness to the next stage of cannabis as it breaks through the prohibition period of the past and is thrust back into the medical industry, now armed with a new level of technology to help amplify its impact and reach.

Thank you for reading this book and taking the time to learn about this ancient medicine. For patients I hope this book has been easy to follow and delivers an understanding of the basic aspects of cannabis medicine and for doctors I hope to have inspired you to take action to help those suffering patients you know may benefit from its various therapeutic properties.

References

Section 1 | The Basics

1. National Academies of Sciences, Engineering, and Medicine. The Health Effects of Cannabis and Cannabinoids: The Current State of Evidence and Recommendations for Research. Washington: The National Academies Press; 2017:85-128. doi: https://doi.org/10.17226/24625.

2. Piomelli D, Russo EB. The Cannabis sativa Versus Cannabis indica Debate: An Interview with Ethan Russo, MD. Cannabis Cannabinoid Res. 2016;1(1):44–46. Published 2016 Jan 1. doi:10.1089/can.2015.29003.ebr

3. Atakan Z. Cannabis, a complex plant: different compounds and different effects on individuals. Therapeutic Advances in Psychopharmacology. 2012 Sep;2(6):241-254. Doi:10.1177/2045125312457586.

4. Cervantes J. The Cannabis Encyclopedia: The Definitive Guide to Cultivation & Consumption of Medical Marijuana. USA: Van Patten Publishing; 2015. ISBN: 1-878823-34-5

5. McPartland J, Russo EB. Cannabis and Cannabis Extracts: Greater Than the Sum of Their Parts? Journal of Cannabis Therapeutics. 2001;1(3-4):103-132. Doi: 10.1300/J175v01n03_08

6. Sinclair J. An introduction to cannabis and the endocannabinoid system. Australian Journal of Herbal Medicine. 2016;28(4):107-125. Available at: https://search.informit.com.au/documentSummary;dn=484958787162768;res=IELHEA.

7. De Petrocellis L, Di Marzo V. An introduction to the endocannabinoid system: From the early to the latest concepts. Best Practice & Research Clinical Endocrinology & Metabolism. 2009;23(1):1-15. Doi: https://doi.org/10.1016/j.beem.2008.10.013.

8. Pertwee RG. Cannabinoid pharmacology: the first 66 years. Br J Pharmacol. 2006;147 Suppl 1(Suppl 1):S163–S171. doi:10.1038/sj.bjp.0706406

9. National Academies of Sciences, Engineering, and Medicine. The Health Effects of Cannabis and Cannabinoids: The Current State of Evidence and Recommendations for Research. Washington: The National Academies Press; 2017:85-128. doi: https://doi.org/10.17226/24625.

10. Lu H-C, Mackie K. An introduction to the endogenous cannabinoid system. Biological psychiatry. 2016;79(7):516-525. doi: https://doi.org/10.1016/j.biopsych.2015.07.028.

11. McPartland JM, Guy GW, Di Marzo V. Care and Feeding of the Endocannabinoid System: A Systematic Review of Potential Clinical Interventions that Upregulate the Endocannabinoid System. Romanovsky AA, ed. PLoS ONE. 2014;9(3):e89566. doi: https://doi.org/10.1371/journal.pone.0089566.

12. Kendall DA, Yudowski GA. Cannabinoid Receptors in the Central Nervous System: Their Signaling and Roles in Disease. Frontiers in Cellular Neuroscience. 2016;10:294. doi:10.3389/fncel.2016.00294.

McPartland JM, Duncan M, Di Marzo V, Pertwee RG. Are cannabidiol and Δ9-tetrahydrocannabivarin negative modulators of the endocannabinoid system? A systematic review. British Journal of Pharmacology. 2015;172(3):737-753. doi:10.1111/bph.12944.

13. McPartland JM, Duncan M, Di Marzo V, Pertwee RG. Are cannabidiol and Δ9-tetrahydrocannabivarin negative modulators of the endocannabinoid system? A systematic review. British Journal of Pharmacology. 2015;172(3):737-753. doi:10.1111/bph.12944.

14. Atakan Z. Cannabis, a complex plant: different compounds and different effects on individuals. Therapeutic Advances in Psychopharmacology. 2012;2(6):241-254. doi: https://doi.org/10.1177/2045125312457586.

15. Mandal A. Cannabinoid Receptors. News Medical: Life Sciences. Feb, 2019 https://www.news-medical.net/health/Cannabinoid-Receptors.aspx.

16. Turcotte C, Blanchet M-R, Laviolette M, Flamand N. The CB2 receptor and its role as a regulator of inflammation. Cellular and Molecular Life Sciences. 2016;73(23):4449-4470. doi:10.1007/s00018-016-2300-4.

17. McPartland JM, Blanchon D, Musty R. CLINICAL STUDY: Cannabimimetic effects modulated by cholinergic compounds. Addiction Biology. 2008;13(3□4):411-415. Doi: 10.1111/j.1369-1600.2008.00126.x

18. Di Marzo V, De Petrocellis L, Fezza F, Ligresti A, Bisogno T. Anandamide receptors. Prostaglandins, Leukotrienes and Essential Fatty Acids (PLEFA). 2002; 66(2–3):377-391. doi: 10.1054/plef.2001.0349.

19. Reggio PH. Endocannabinoid binding to the cannabinoid receptors: what is known and what remains unknown. Curr Med Chem. 2010;17(14):1468–1486.

20. Ahn K, McKinney MK, Cravatt BF. Enzymatic Pathways That Regulate Endocannabinoid Signaling in the Nervous System. Chemical reviews. 2008;108(5):1687-1707. doi: https://doi.org/10.1021/cr0782067.

21. Alger BE, Kim J. Supply and demand for endocannabinoids. Trends in neurosciences. 2011;34(6):304-315. doi:10.1016/j.tins.2011.03.003.

22. Griffing GT. Endocannabinoids. Medscape. 2018. https://emedicine.

medscape.com/article/1361971.
23. Goldstein B. The Endocannabinoid System. 2015. Available at: http://weedmaps-marketing.squarespace.com/articles/2015/9/20/the-endocannabinoid-system.
24. Pleuvry, B. Receptors, agonists and antagonists. Anaesthesia & Intensive Care Medicine. 2004;5(10), 350-352. Doi: https://doi.org/10.1383/anes.5.10.350.52312.
25. Nussinov R, Tsai C. The Different Ways through Which Specificity Works in Orthosteric and Allosteric Drugs. Current Pharmaceutical Design. 2012;18(9):1311-1316. Doi: 10.2174/138161212799436377.
26. Pertwee RG. The diverse CB1 and CB2 receptor pharmacology of three plant cannabinoids: Δ9-tetrahydrocannabinol, cannabidiol and Δ9-tetrahydrocannabivarin. British Journal of Pharmacology. 2008;153(2):199-215. doi:10.1038/sj.bjp.0707442.
27. Martínez-Pinilla E, Varani K, Reyes-Resina I, et al. Binding and Signaling Studies Disclose a Potential Allosteric Site for Cannabidiol in Cannabinoid CB2 Receptors. Frontiers in Pharmacology. 2017;8:744. doi:10.3389/fphar.2017.00744.
28. Sullivan JM, Schweizer FE. Neurotransmitter Release from Presynaptic Terminals. In: eLS. John Wiley & Sons Ltd, Chichester. 2015. doi: https://doi.org/10.1002/9780470015902.a0000285.pub2.
29. Placzek EA, Okamoto Y, Ueda N, Barker EL. Mechanisms for Recycling and Biosynthesis of Endogenous Cannabinoids Anandamide and 2-Arachidonylglycerol. Journal of neurochemistry. 2008;107(4):987-1000. doi: https://doi.org/10.1111/j.1471-4159.2008.05659.x.
30. Atakan Z. Cannabis, a complex plant: different compounds and different effects on individuals. Therapeutic Advances in Psychopharmacology. 2012;2(6):241-254. doi: https://doi.org/10.1177/2045125312457586.

Section 2 | Pharmacology

1. Sinclair J. An introduction to cannabis and the endocannabinoid system. Australian Journal of Herbal Medicine. 2016;28(4):107-125.
2. Kendall DA, Yudowski GA. Cannabinoid Receptors in the Central Nervous System: Their Signaling and Roles in Disease. Frontiers in Cellular Neuroscience. 2016;10:294. Doi: https://doi.org/10.3389/fncel.2016.00294
3. NIDA. Letter From the Director. (2018, February 12). Marijuana.

Retrieved from https://www.drugabuse.gov/publications/research-reports/marijuana.

4. Russo EB, Hohmann AG. Role of Cannabinoids in Pain Management. In: Deer T. et al. (eds) Comprehensive Treatment of Chronic Pain by Medical, Interventional, and Integrative Approaches. Springer, New York, NY; 2013:181-197. Doi: https://doi.org/10.1007/978-1-4614-1560-2_18.

5. The Science of the Endocannabinoid System: How THC Affects the Brain and the Body. 2011. Available at: http://headsup.scholastic.com/students/endocannabinoid. Accessed March 10, 2018.

6. Nagarkatti P, Pandey R, Rieder SA, Hegde VL, Nagarkatti M. Cannabinoids as novel anti-inflammatory drugs. Future medicinal chemistry. 2009;1(7):1333-1349. Doi: https://doi.org/10.4155/fmc.09.93.

7. Russo EB. Cannabinoids in the management of difficult to treat pain. Ther Clin Risk Manag. 2008;4(1):245–259.

8. Sharkey KA, Darmani NA, Parker LA. Regulation of nausea and vomiting by cannabinoids and the endocannabinoid system. European journal of pharmacology. 2014;722:10.1016/j.ejphar.2013.09.068. Doi: https://doi.org/10.1016/j.ejphar.2013.09.068.

9. Parker LA, Rock EM, Limebeer CL. Regulation of nausea and vomiting by cannabinoids. British Journal of Pharmacology. 2011;163(7):1411-1422. Doi: https://doi.org/10.1111/j.1476-5381.2010.01176.x.

10. Gamage TF, Lichtman AH. The Endocannabinoid System: Role in Energy Regulation. Pediatric blood & cancer. 2012;58(1):144-148. Doi: https://doi.org/10.1002/pbc.23367.

11. Rosenberg EC, Tsien RW, Whalley BJ, Devinsky O. Cannabinoids and Epilepsy. Neurotherapeutics. 2015;12(4):747-768. doi: https://doi.org/10.1007/s13311-015-0375-5.

12. Guzmán, M, Duarte, M J, Blázquez, C, Ravina, J, Rosa, M C, Galve-Roperh, I, Sánchez, C, Velasco, G. A pilot clinical study of Δ9-tetrahydrocannabinol in patients with recurrent glioblastoma multiforme. British Journal of Cancer. 2006;95: 197–203. doi: https://doi.org/10.1111/j.1749-6632.2000.tb06193.x.

13. Hampson AJ, Grimaldi M, Lolic M, Wink D, Rosenthal R, Axelrod J. Neuroprotective Antioxidants from Marijuana. Annals of the New York Academy of Sciences. 2000;899: 274–282. doi: https://doi.org/10.1111/j.1749-6632.2000.tb06193.x.

14. World Health Organisation. CANNABIDIOL (CBD) Pre-Review Report Agenda Item 5.2 http://www.who.int/medicines/access/controlled-substances/5.2_CBD.pdf.

15. Martínez-Pinilla E, Varani K, Reyes-Resina I, et al. Binding and

Signaling Studies Disclose a Potential Allosteric Site for Cannabidiol in Cannabinoid CB2 Receptors. Frontiers in Pharmacology. 2017;8:744. Doi: https://doi.org/10.3389/fphar.2017.00744.

16. Elmes MW, Kaczocha M, Berger WT, et al. Fatty Acid-binding Proteins (FABPs) Are Intracellular Carriers for Δ9-Tetrahydrocannabinol (THC) and Cannabidiol (CBD). The Journal of Biological Chemistry. 2015;290(14):8711-8721. doi: https://doi.org/10.1074/jbc.M114.618447.

17. Costa B, Giagnoni G, Franke C, Trovato AE, Colleoni M. Vanilloid TRPV1 receptor mediates the antihyperalgesic effect of the nonpsychoactive cannabinoid, cannabidiol, in a rat model of acute inflammation. British Journal of Pharmacology. 2004;143(2):247-250. doi: https://doi.org/10.1038/sj.bjp.0705920.

18. Ibeas Bih C, Chen T, Nunn AVW, Bazelot M, Dallas M, Whalley BJ. Molecular Targets of Cannabidiol in Neurological Disorders. Neurotherapeutics. 2015;12(4):699-730. doi: https://doi.org/10.1007/s13311-015-0377-3.

19. Xiong W, Cui T, Cheng K, et al. Cannabinoids suppress inflammatory and neuropathic pain by targeting α3 glycine receptors. The Journal of Experimental Medicine. 2012;209(6):1121-1134. doi: https://doi.org/10.1084/jem.20120242.

20. Iffland K, Grotenhermen F. An Update on Safety and Side Effects of Cannabidiol: A Review of Clinical Data and Relevant Animal Studies. Cannabis and Cannabinoid Research. 2017;2(1):139-154. doi: https://doi.org/10.1089/can.2016.0034.

21. Cechova S, Elsobky AM, Venton BJ. A1 receptors self-regulate adenosine release in the striatum: evidence of autoreceptor characteristics. Neuroscience. 2010;171(4):1006-1015. doi: https://doi.org/10.1016/j.neuroscience.2010.09.063.

22. Prud'homme M, Cata R, Jutras-Aswad D. Cannabidiol as an Intervention for Addictive Behaviors: A Systematic Review of the Evidence. Substance Abuse: Research and Treatment. 2015;9:33-38. doi: https://doi.org/10.4137/SART.S25081.

23. Alger BE. Endocannabinoids and Their Implications for Epilepsy. Epilepsy Currents. 2004;4(5):169-173. doi: https://doi.org/10.1111/j.1535-7597.2004.04501.x.

24. Likar R, Nahler G. The use of cannabis in supportive care and treatment of brain tumor. Neuro-Oncology Practice. 2017;4(3):151-160. Doi: https://doi.org/10.1093/nop/npw027.

25. Ren Y, Whittard J, Higuera-Matas A, Morris CV, Hurd YL.

110

Cannabidiol, a nonpsychotropic component of cannabis, inhibits cue-induced heroin-seeking and normalises discrete mesolimbic neuronal disturbances. The Journal of neuroscience: the official journal of the Society for Neuroscience. 2009;29(47):14764-14769. doi: https://doi.org/10.1523/JNEUROSCI.4291-09.2009.

26. Lee MA. How CBD Works. 2016. Available at: https://greenflowerbotanicals.com/how-cbd-works/. Accessed March 22, 2018.

27. Sugaya Y, Yamazaki M, Uchigashima M, et al. Crucial Roles of the Endocannabinoid 2-Arachidonoylglycerol in the Suppression of Epileptic Seizures. Cell Reports. 2016;16(5):1405-1415. Doi: https://doi.org/10.1016/j.celrep.2016.06.083.

28. Whyte LS, Ryberg E, Sims NA, et al. The putative cannabinoid receptor GPR55 affects osteoclast function in vitro and bone mass in vivo. Proceedings of the National Academy of Sciences of the United States of America. 2009;106(38):16511-16516. doi: https://doi.org/10.1073/pnas.0902743106.

29. Andradas C, Caffarel MM, Pérez-Gómez E, et al. The orphan G protein-coupled receptor GPR55 promotes cancer cell proliferation via ERK. Oncogene, 2010;30(2):245-52. Doi: https://doi.org/10.1038/onc.2010.402.

30. McAllister SD, Christian RT, Horowitz MP, Garcia A, Desprez P. Cannabidiol as a novel inhibitor of Id-1 gene expression in aggressive breast cancer cells. American Association for Cancer Research. 2007;6(11):2921-2927. Doi: https://doi.org/10.1158/1535-7163.MCT-07-0371.

31. O'Sullivan SE. An update on PPAR activation by cannabinoids. British Journal of Pharmacology. 2016;173(12):1899-1910. doi: https://doi.org/10.1111/bph.13497.

32. National Cancer Institute. Cannabis and Cannabinoids (PDQ®)–Health Professional Version. 2017. Availalble at: https://www.cancer.gov/about-cancer/treatment/cam/hp/cannabis-pdq. Accessed April 16, 2018.

33. Ripley E. Medicinal Value of Cannabinol (CBN). Medical Marijuana, Inc. 2018 [cited 15 May 2018]. Available from: https://www.medicalmarijuanainc.com/medicinal-value-of-cannabinol-cbn/.

34. What is CBC (Cannabichromene)? [Internet]. Leaf Science. 2018 [cited 15 May 2018]. Available from: https://www.leafscience.com/2017/05/07/what-is-cbc-cannabichromene/.

35. What is CBG (Cannabigerol)? [Internet]. Leaf Science. 2018 [cited 15 May 2018]. Available from: https://www.leafscience.com/2017/04/26/what-is-cbg-cannabigerol/.

36. Hartsel A J, Eades J, Hickory B, Makriyannis A. Cannabis sativa and Hemp. Nutraceuticals Efficacy, Safety & Toxicity. 2016:735-754. Doi: https://doi.org/10.1016/B978-0-12-802147-7.00053-X

37. MacCallum CA1, Russo EB. Practical considerations in medical cannabis administration and dosing. Eur J Intern Med. 2018 Mar;49:12-19. doi: 10.1016/j.ejim.2018.01.004.

38. Russo EB. Clinical endocannabinoid deficiency (CECD): can this concept explain therapeutic benefits of cannabis in migraine, fibromyalgia, irritable bowel syndrome and other treatment-resistant conditions? Neuro Endocrinol Letters. 2008;29(2):192-200. Available at: https://www.ncbi.nlm.nih.gov/pubmed/18404144.

39. Goldstein B. The Best Offense: Preventive Medicine Gains an Ally in Cannabis. 2017. Available at: https://health.usnews.com/health-care/for-better/articles/2017-12-29/the-best-offense-preventive-medicine-gains-an-ally-in-cannabis.

40. Andre CM, Hausman J-F, Guerriero G. Cannabis sativa: The Plant of the Thousand and One Molecules. Frontiers in Plant Science. 2016;7:19. Doi: https://doi.org/10.3389/fpls.2016.00019.

41. Du Plessis SS, Agarwal A, Syriac A. Marijuana, phytocannabinoids, the endocannabinoid system, and male fertility. Journal of Assisted Reproduction and Genetics. 2015;32(11):1575-1588. Doi: https://doi.org/10.1007/s10815-015-0553-8.

42. McPartland JM, Duncan M, Di Marzo V, Pertwee RG. Are cannabidiol and Δ9-tetrahydrocannabivarin negative modulators of the endocannabinoid system? A systematic review. British Journal of Pharmacology. 2015;172(3):737-753. Doi: https://doi.org/10.1111/bph.12944.

43. DeFalco L. The Major Role of Minor Cannabinoids. 2018. Available at: https://www.cb1cap.com/major-role-minor-cannabinoids/. Accessed March 31, 2018.

44. Grotenhermen F. Pharmacology of cannabinoids. Neuro Endocrinology Letters. 2004;25(1-2):14-23. Available at: https://www.ncbi.nlm.nih.gov/pubmed/15159677.

45. Huff J, Chan P. Antitumor effects of THC. Environmental Health Perspectives. 2000;108(10):A442-A443. Available at: https://www.ncbi.nlm.nih.gov/pmc/articles/PMC1240145/.

46. Sharkey KA, Darmani NA, Parker LA. Regulation of nausea and vomiting by cannabinoids and the endocannabinoid system. European journal of pharmacology. 2014;722:10.1016/j.ejphar.2013.09.068. doi:10.1016/j.ejphar.2013.09.068.

47. Parker LA, Rock EM, Limebeer CL. Regulation of nausea
and vomiting by cannabinoids. British Journal of Pharmacology.
2011;163(7):1411-1422. doi:10.1111/j.1476-5381.2010.01176.x.
48. National Academies of Sciences, Engineering, and Medicine. The
Health Effects of Cannabis and Cannabinoids: The Current State of
Evidence and Recommendations for Research. Washington: The National
Academies Press; 2017:85-128. doi: https://doi.org/10.17226/24625.

Section 3 | Clinical Applications

1. Bupa. Chronic Pain Fact Sheet. 2011. Available at: https://www.bupa.
com.au/health-and-wellness/health-information/az-health-information/
chronic-pain-fact-sheet.
2. Finan PH, Smith MT. The Comorbidity of Insomnia, Chronic Pain, and
Depression: Dopamine as a Putative Mechanism. Sleep medicine reviews.
2013;17(3):173-183. Doi: https://doi.org/10.1016/j.smrv.2012.03.003.
3. National Academies of Sciences, Engineering, and Medicine. The
Health Effects of Cannabis and Cannabinoids: The Current State of
Evidence and Recommendations for Research. Washington: The National
Academies Press; 2017:85-128. doi: https://doi.org/10.17226/24625.
4. Zettl UK, Rommer P, Hipp P, Patejdl R. Evidence for the efficacy and
effectiveness of THC-CBD oromucosal spray in symptom management
of patients with spasticity due to multiple sclerosis. Therapeutic
Advances in Neurological Disorders. 2016;9(1):9-30. Doi: https://doi.
org/10.1177/1756285615612659.
5. Blake A, Wan B, Malek L, et al. A selective review of medical cannabis
in cancer pain management. Annals of Palliative Medicine. 2017;6(Suppl
2):S215-S222. Doi: https://doi.org/10.21037/apm.2017.08.05.
6. Ibeas Bih C, Chen T, Nunn AVW, Bazelot M, Dallas M, Whalley
BJ. Molecular Targets of Cannabidiol in Neurological Disorders.
Neurotherapeutics. 2015;12(4):699-730. doi: https://doi.org/10.1007/
s13311-015-0377-3.
7. World Health Organization. CANNABIDIOL (CBD) Pre-Review
Report Agenda Item 5.2 http://www.who.int/medicines/access/
controlled-substances/5.2_CBD.pdf.
8. Xiong W, Cui T, Cheng K, et al. Cannabinoids suppress inflammatory
and neuropathic pain by targeting α3 glycine receptors. The Journal
of Experimental Medicine. 2012;209(6):1121-1134. doi: https://doi.
org/10.1084/jem.20120242.
9. Boehnke KF, Litinas E, Clauw DJ, et al. Medical Cannabis Use Is

Associated With Decreased Opiate Medication Use in a Retrospective Cross-Sectional Survey of Patients With Chronic Pain. The Journal of Pain. 17(6):739-744. DOI: https://doi.org/10.1016/j.jpain.2016.03.002.

10. Prud'homme M, Cata R, Jutras-Aswad D. Cannabidiol as an Intervention for Addictive Behaviors: A Systematic Review of the Evidence. Substance Abuse: Research and Treatment. 2015;9:33-38. doi: https://doi.org/10.4137/SART.S25081.

11. Monheit B, Pietrzak D, Hocking S. Prescription drug abuse - A timely update. Australian Family Physician. 2016;45(12):862-866. Available at: https://www.racgp.org.au/afp/2016/december/prescription-drug-abuse-a-timely-update/.

12. Humphreys K. Avoiding globalisation of the prescription opioid epidemic. The Lancet. 2017;390(10093):437-439. Doi: https://doi.org/10.1016/S0140-6736(17)31918-9.

13. Bachhuber MA, Saloner B, Cunningham CO, Barry CL. Medical cannabis laws and opioid analgesic overdose mortality in the United States, 1999-2010. JAMA Internal Medicine. 2014;174(10):1668-1673. doi: https://doi.org/10.1001/jamainternmed.2014.4005.

14. Ren Y, Whittard J, Higuera-Matas A, Morris CV, Hurd YL. Cannabidiol, a non-psychotropic component of cannabis, inhibits cue-induced heroin-seeking and normalizes discrete mesolimbic neuronal disturbances. The Journal of neuroscience: the official journal of the Society for Neuroscience. 2009;29(47):14764-14769. doi: https://doi.org/10.1523/JNEUROSCI.4291-09.2009.

15. Iffland K, Grotenhermen F. An Update on Safety and Side Effects of Cannabidiol: A Review of Clinical Data and Relevant Animal Studies. Cannabis and Cannabinoid Research. 2017;2(1):139-154. doi: https://doi.org/10.1089/can.2016.0034.

16. Elmes MW, Kaczocha M, Berger WT, et al. Fatty Acid-binding Proteins (FABPs) Are Intracellular Carriers for Δ9-Tetrahydrocannabinol (THC) and Cannabidiol (CBD). The Journal of Biological Chemistry. 2015;290(14):8711-8721. doi: https://doi.org/10.1074/jbc.M114.618447.

17. Costa B, Giagnoni G, Franke C, Trovato AE, Colleoni M. Vanilloid TRPV1 receptor mediates the antihyperalgesic effect of the non-psychoactive cannabinoid, cannabidiol, in a rat model of acute inflammation. British Journal of Pharmacology. 2004;143(2):247-250. doi: https://doi.org/10.1038/sj.bjp.0705920.

18. Cechova S, Elsobky AM, Venton BJ. A1 receptors self-regulate adenosine release in the striatum: evidence of autoreceptor characteristics. Neuroscience. 2010;171(4):1006-1015. doi: https://doi.org/10.1016/j.

neuroscience.2010.09.063.
19. Nielsen S, Sabioni P, Trigo JM, et al. Opioid-Sparing Effect of Cannabinoids: A Systematic Review and Meta-Analysis. Neuropsychopharmacology. 2017;42(9):1752–1765. doi:10.1038/npp.2017.51
20. NCI. Cannabis and Cannabinoids (PDQ®)–Health Professional Version. https://www.cancer.gov/about-cancer/treatment/cam/hp/cannabis-pdq. Updated Jan, 2019.
21. Śledziński P, Zeyland J, Słomski R, Nowak A. The current state and future perspectives of cannabinoids in cancer biology [published correction appears in Cancer Med. 2018 Nov;7(11):5859]. Cancer Med. 2018;7(3):765–775. doi:10.1002/cam4.1312
22. Sharafi G, He H, Nikfarjam M. Potential Use of Cannabinoids for the Treatment of Pancreatic Cancer. J Pancreatic Cancer. 2019;5(1):1–7. Published 2019 Jan 25. doi:10.1089/pancan.2018.0019
23. O'Sullivan SE. An update on PPAR activation by cannabinoids. Br J Pharmacol. 2016;173(12):1899–1910. doi:10.1111/bph.13497
24. Gandhi S, Vasisth G, Kapoor A. Systematic review of the potential role of cannabinoids as antiproliferative agents for urological cancers. Can Urol Assoc J. 2017;11(3-4):E138–E142. doi:10.5489/cuaj.4371
25. Casanova ML, Blázquez C, Martínez-Palacio J, et al. Inhibition of skin tumor growth and angiogenesis in vivo by activation of cannabinoid receptors. J Clin Invest. 2003;111(1):43–50. doi:10.1172/JCI16116
26. Cohen L, de Moor CA, Eisenberg P, Ming EE, Hu H. Chemotherapy-induced nausea and vomiting: incidence and impact on patient quality of life at community oncology settings. Support Care Cancer. 2007 May;15(5):497-503. Doi: 10.1007/s00520-006-0173-z
27. Burke TA1, Wisniewski T, Ernst FR. Resource utilization and costs associated with chemotherapy-induced nausea and vomiting (CINV) following highly or moderately emetogenic chemotherapy administered in the US outpatient hospital setting. Supportive care in cancer: official journal of the Multinational Association of Supportive Care in Cancer. 2011 Jan;19(1):131-40. doi: 10.1007/s00520-009-0797-x.
28. Janelsins MC, Tejani MA, Kamen C, Peoples AR, Mustian KM, Morrow GR. Current pharmacotherapy for chemotherapy-induced nausea and vomiting in cancer patients. Expert Opin Pharmacother. 2013;14(6):757–766. doi:10.1517/14656566.2013.776541
29. Sharkey KA, Darmani NA, Parker LA. Regulation of nausea and vomiting by cannabinoids and the endocannabinoid system. European journal of pharmacology. 2014;722. doi: https://doi.org/10.1016/j.

ejphar.2013.09.068.

30. May MB, Glode AE. Dronabinol for chemotherapy-induced nausea and vomiting unresponsive to antiemetics. Cancer Management and Research. 2016;8:49-55. doi:10.2147/CMAR.S81425.

31. Smith LA, Azariah F, Lavender VTC, Stoner NS, Bettiol S. Cannabinoids for nausea and vomiting in adults with cancer receiving chemotherapy. Cochrane Database of Systematic Reviews. 2015;(11). DOI: https://doi.org/10.1002/14651858.CD009464.pub2.

32. Parker L, Rock E, Limebeer C. Regulation of nausea and vomiting by cannabinoids. British Journal of Pharmacology. 2011;163(7):1411-1422. Doi: https://doi.org/10.1111/j.1476-5381.2010.01176.x.

33. Rock EM, Parker LA. Cannabinoids as Potential Treatment for Chemotherapy-Induced Nausea and Vomiting. Doi: https://doi.org/10.3389/fphar.2016.00221.

34. Abrams DI. Integrating cannabis into clinical cancer care. Current Oncology. 2016;23(Suppl 2):S8-S14. Doi: https://doi.org/10.3747/co.23.3099.

35. National Academies of Sciences, Engineering, and Medicine. The health effects of cannabis and cannabinoids: Current state of evidence and recommendations for research. Washington, DC: The National Academies Press. 2017.

36. Aggarwal SK. Use of cannabinoids in cancer care: palliative care. Current Oncology. 2016;23(Suppl 2):S33-S36. doi:10.3747/co.23.2962. Available at: https://www.ncbi.nlm.nih.gov/pmc/articles/PMC4791145/.

37. World Health Organization. WHO Definition of Palliative Care. 2018. Available at: http://www.who.int/cancer/palliative/definition/en/.

38. Benyamin R, Trescot AM, Datta S, et al. Opioid complications and side effects. Pain Physician, 2008;11(2 Suppl), S105-20. Available at: https://www.ncbi.nlm.nih.gov/pubmed/18443635.

39. Pertwee RG. The diverse CB1 and CB2 receptor pharmacology of three plant cannabinoids: Δ9-tetrahydrocannabinol, cannabidiol and Δ9-tetrahydrocannabivarin. British Journal of Pharmacology. 2008;153(2):199-215. doi: https://doi.org/10.1038/sj.bjp.0707442.

40. Mack A, Joy J. Marijuana as medicine? The science beyond the controversy. 2000. Available at: https://www.nap.edu/catalog/9586/marijuana-as-medicine-the-science-beyond-the-controversy.

41. University of Buffalo. RIA neuroscience study points to possible use of medical marijuana for depression. 2015. Available at: http://www.buffalo.edu/news/releases/2015/02/004.html.

42. Wiese B, Wilson-Poe AR. Emerging Evidence for Cannabis' Role in Opioid Use Disorder. Cannabis Cannabinoid Res. 2018;3(1):179–189. Published 2018 Sep 1. doi:10.1089/can.2018.0022

43. Rosenberg EC, Tsien RW, Whalley BJ, Devinsky O. Cannabinoids and Epilepsy. Neurotherapeutics. 2015;12(4):747-768. doi:10.1007/s13311-015-0375-5.

44. Turkanis SA, Smiley KA, Borys HK, Olsen DM, Karler R. An Electrophysiological Analysis of the Anticonvulsant Action of Cannabidiol on Limbic Seizures in Conscious Rats. Epilepsia. 1979;20(4):351-363. Doi: https://doi.org/10.1111/j.1528-1157.1979.tb04815.x.

45. Kolikonda MK, Srinivasan K, Enja M, et al. Medical Marijuana for Epilepsy? Innovations in Clinical Neuroscience. 2016;13(3-4):23-26. Available at: https://www.ncbi.nlm.nih.gov/pmc/articles/PMC4911937/.

46. Veldhuis WB, Van Der Stelt M, Wadman MW, et al. Neuroprotection by the Endogenous Cannabinoid Anandamide and Arvanil against In Vivo Excitotoxicity in the Rat: Role of Vanilloid Receptors and Lipoxygenases. Journal of Neuroscience. 2003;23(10):4127-4133. Available at: https://www.ncbi.nlm.nih.gov/pubmed/12764100.

47. Al-Hayani A. Anticonvulsant action of anandamide in an in vitro model of epilepsy. Neurosciences (Riyadh, Saudi Arabia). 2005;10(3):205-209. Available at: https://www.ncbi.nlm.nih.gov/pubmed/22473259.

48. Colizzi M, Mcguire P, Pertwee RG, Bhattacharyya S. Effect of cannabis on glutamate signalling in the brain: A systematic review of human and animal evidence. Neuroscience and Biobehavioral Reviews. 2016;64:359-381. Doi: https://doi.org/10.1016/j.neubiorev.2016.03.010.

49. Malfitano AM, Proto MC, Bifulco M. Cannabinoids in the management of spasticity associated with multiple sclerosis. Neuropsychiatric Disease and Treatment. 2008;4(5):847-853. Available at: https://www.ncbi.nlm.nih.gov/pmc/articles/PMC2626929/.

50. Malfitano AM, Matarese G, Bifulco M. From cannabis to endocannabinoids in multiple sclerosis: a paradigm of central nervous system autoimmune diseases. Curr Drug Targets CNS Neurol Disord. 2005;4(6):667-75. Available at: https://www.ncbi.nlm.nih.gov/pubmed/16375684.

51. Fernández-Ruiz J, Sagredo O, Pazos MR, et al. Cannabidiol for neurodegenerative disorders: important new clinical applications for this phytocannabinoid?. Br J Clin Pharmacol. 2012;75(2):323–333. doi:10.1111/j.1365-2125.2012.04341.x

52. Iuvone T, Esposito G, De Filippis D, Scuderi C, Steardo L. Cannabidiol: A Promising Drug for Neurodegenerative Disorders?

CNS Neuroscience & Therapeutics. 2009;15(1):65-75. Doi: https://doi.org/10.1111/j.1755-5949.2008.00065.x.

53. Parkinson's Disease: Cannabinoids and CBD Research Overview. 2017. Available at: https://echoconnection.org/parkinsons-disease-medical-cannabis-and-cbd-research-overview/. Accessed March 24, 2018.

54. Tambaro S, Bortolato M. Cannabinoid-related agents in the treatment of anxiety disorders: current knowledge and future perspectives. Recent patents on CNS drug discovery. 2012;7(1):25-40. Available at: https://www.ncbi.nlm.nih.gov/pmc/articles/PMC3691841/.

55. Cao, C., Liu, H., & Lin, X. The Potential Therapeutic Effects of THC on Alzheimers Disease. Journal of Alzheimer's Disease, 2014;42(3):973-984. Available at: https://www.ncbi.nlm.nih.gov/pubmed/25024327.

56. Universität Bonn. 2017. Cannabis reverses ageing processes in the brain. Available at: https://www.uni-bonn.de/news/128-2017. Accessed March 24, 2018.

57. More SV, Choi D-K. Promising cannabinoid-based therapies for Parkinson's disease: motor symptoms to neuroprotection. Molecular Neurodegeneration. 2015;10:17. Doi: https://doi.org/10.1186/s13024-015-0012-0.

58. IDF (International Diabetes Federation). IDF Diabetes Atlas 7th Edition (2015). Available: https://www.idf.org/e-library/epidemiology-research/diabetes-atlas/13-diabetes-atlas-seventh-edition.html

59. Penner EA1, Buettner H, Mittleman MA. The impact of marijuana use on glucose, insulin, and insulin resistance among US adults. Am J Med. 2013 Jul;126(7):583-9. doi: 10.1016/j.amjmed.2013.03.002.

60. Liou GI. Diabetic retinopathy: Role of inflammation and potential therapies for anti-inflammation. World J Diabetes. 2010;1(1):12–18. doi:10.4239/wjd.v1.i1.12

61. Nagarkatti P, Pandey R, Rieder SA, Hegde VL, Nagarkatti M. Cannabinoids as novel anti-inflammatory drugs. Future Med Chem. 2009;1(7):1333–1349. doi:10.4155/fmc.09.93

62. Russo EB. Cannabinoids in the management of difficult to treat pain. Ther Clin Risk Manag. 2008;4(1):245–259.

63. Otten R, Engels RC. Testing bidirectional effects between cannabis use and depressive symptoms: moderation by the serotonin transporter gene. Addict Biol. 2013 Sep;18(5):826-35. doi: 10.1111/j.1369-1600.2011.00380.x.

64. Krystal JH, Neumeister A. Noradrenergic and serotonergic mechanisms in the neurobiology of posttraumatic stress disorder and resilience. Brain Res. 2009;1293:13–23. doi:10.1016/j.brainres.2009.03.044

65. Williamson JB, Porges EC, Lamb DG, Porges SW. Maladaptive autonomic regulation in PTSD accelerates physiological aging. Front Psychol. 2015;5:1571. Published 2015 Jan 21. doi:10.3389/fpsyg.2014.01571

66. Krystal JH, Abdallah CG, Averill LA, et al. Synaptic Loss and the Pathophysiology of PTSD: Implications for Ketamine as a Prototype Novel Therapeutic. Curr Psychiatry Rep. 2017;19(10):74. Published 2017 Aug 26. doi:10.1007/s11920-017-0829-z

67. Roy-Byrne P. Cannabinoid System Dysregulation in PTSD. Jun 2013. Available: https://www.jwatch.org/na31258/2013/06/10/cannabinoid-system-dysregulation-ptsd

68. US DVA. PTSD and Substance Abuse in Veterans. Updated 2019. https://www.ptsd.va.gov/understand/related/substance_abuse_vet.asp

69. Prud'homme M, Cata R, Jutras-Aswad D. Cannabidiol as an Intervention for Addictive Behaviors: A Systematic Review of the Evidence. Subst Abuse. 2015;9:33–38. Published 2015 May 21. doi:10.4137/SART.S25081

70. Shishko I, Oliveira R, Moore TA, Almeida K. A review of medical marijuana for the treatment of posttraumatic stress disorder: Real symptom re-leaf or just high hopes?. Ment Health Clin. 2018;8(2):86–94. Published 2018 Mar 26. doi:10.9740/mhc.2018.03.086

71. IOF (International Osteoporosis Foundation). EPIDEMIOLOGY. https://www.iofbonehealth.org/epidemiology. 2017.

72. AIHW. Estimating the prevalence of osteoporosis in Australia. https://www.aihw.gov.au/reports/chronic-musculoskeletal-conditions/estimating-the-prevalence-of-osteoporosis-in-austr/contents/summary. 2014.

73. Idris AI. Cannabinoid receptors as target for treatment of osteoporosis: a tale of two therapies. Curr Neuropharmacol. 2010;8(3):243–253. doi:10.2174/157015910792246173

74. Elefteriou F, Campbell P, Ma Y. Control of bone remodeling by the peripheral sympathetic nervous system. Calcif Tissue Int. 2013;94(1):140–151. doi:10.1007/s00223-013-9752-4

75. Bab I, Zimmer A, Melamed E. Cannabinoids and the skeleton: from marijuana to reversal of bone loss. Ann Med. 2009;41(8):560-7. doi:10.1080/07853890903121025.

76. Lee A. M. CBD: How It Works. O'Shaughnessy's. https://www.beyondthc.com/wp-content/uploads/2012/08/CBDiary14-15.pdf. Autumn 2011

77. Dutton P Minister For Health. Department of Health Australia -

Antibiotic Awareness Week. http://www.health.gov.au/internet/ministers/publishing.nsf/Content/health-mediarel-yr2014-dutton099.htm. 2014.

78. Kabelik J, Krejci Z and Santavy F. Cannabis as a medicament. U.N. Bulletin on Narcotics. 1960;12(3):5-23. https://www.unodc.org/unodc/en/data-and-analysis/bulletin/bulletin_1960-01-01_3_page003.html

79. Appendino G, Gibbons S, Giana A, Pagani A, Grassi G, Stavri M, Smith E, and Mukhlesur Rahman M. Antibacterial Cannabinoids from Cannabis sativa: A Structure–Activity Study. Journal of Natural Products. 2008;71(8):1427-1430. DOI: 10.1021/np8002673.

80. Hampson AJ, Grimaldi M, Lolic M, Wink D, Rosenthal R, Axelrod J. Neuroprotective Antioxidants from Marijuana. Annals of the New York Academy of Sciences. 2000;899: 274–282. doi: https://doi.org/10.1111/j.1749-6632.2000.tb06193.x

Section 4 | Safety Considerations

1. Therapeutic Goods Administration. Guidance for the use of medicinal cannabis in Australia: Overview. 2017. Available at: https://www.tga.gov.au/publication/guidance-use-medicinal-cannabis-australia-overview. Accessed on 28 March 2018.

2. Maccallum CA, Russo EB. Practical considerations in medical cannabis administration and dosing. European Journal of Internal Medicine. 2018;49:12-19. Doi: https://doi.org/10.1016/j.ejim.2018.01.004.

3. Gable R. Comparison of acute lethal toxicity of commonly abused psychoactive substances. Addiction. 2004;99(6):686-696. Doi: https://doi.org/10.1111/j.1360-0443.2004.00744.x.

4. Gable RS. Comparison of acute lethal toxicity of commonly abused psychoactive substances. Addiction. 2004 Jun;99(6):686-96. DOI: 10.1111/j.1360-0443.2004.00744.x

5. Nutt DJ1, King LA, Phillips LD; Independent Scientific Committee on Drugs. Drug harms in the UK: a multicriteria decision analysis. Lancet. 2010 Nov 6;376(9752):1558-65. doi: 10.1016/S0140-6736(10)61462-6.

6. ABS. Causes of Death, Australia, 2016. https://www.abs.gov.au/ausstats/abs@.nsf/Lookup/by%20Subject/3303.0~2016~Main%20Features~Drug%20Induced%20Deaths%20in%20Australia~6. Updated 2018.

7. Roxburgh, A., and Breen, C. (2016). Accidental drug-induced deaths due to opioids in Australia, 2012. Sydney: National Drug and Alcohol Research Centre, UNSW

8. Roxburgh, A. and Breen, C (2016). Cocaine and methamphetamine

related drug-induced deaths in Australia, 2012. Sydney: National Drug and Alcohol Research Centre, UNSW

Iversen, L. Cannabis and the brain. Brain. 2003;126(6):1252-1270. Doi: https://doi.org/10.1093/brain/awg143.

Hall W, Degenhardt L. Adverse health effects of non-medical cannabis use. Lancet (London, England). 2009;374(9698) 1383-91. Doi: https://doi.org/10.1016/S0140-6736(09)61037-0.

Kalant H. Adverse effects of cannabis on health: An update of the literature since 1996. Progress in Neuro-psychopharmacology & Biological Psychiatry. 2004;28(5):849-63. Doi: https://doi.org/10.1016/j.pnpbp.2004.05.027.

Cannabis/marijuana: what are the effects? Available at: http://www.mydr.com.au/addictions/cannabis-marijuana-what-are-the-effects. Accessed March 28, 2018.

9. Volkow N, Baler R, Compton W, Weiss, S. Adverse Health Effects of Marijuana Use. The New England Journal of Medicine. 2014;370(23):2219-2227. Doi: https://doi.org/10.1056/NEJMra1402309.

10. California Society of Addiction Medicine. The Adverse Effects of Marijuana (for healthcare professionals). Available at: https://www.csam-asam.org/adverse-effects-marijuana-healthcare-professionals. Accessed March 28, 2018.

11. Sun S, Zimmermann AE. Cannabinoid Hyperemesis Syndrome. Hospital Pharmacy. 2013;48(8):650-655. Doi: https://doi.org/10.1310/hpj4808-650.

12. Hartman RL, Brown TL, Milavetz G, et al. Cannabis Effects on Driving Lateral Control With and Without Alcohol. Drug and alcohol dependence. Clinical Chemistry. 2015;154:25-37. doi: https://doi.org/10.1016/j.drugalcdep.2015.06.015.

13. Yamaori S, Koeda K, Kushihara M, et al. Comparison in the In Vitro Inhibitory Effects of Major Phytocannabinoids and Polycyclic Aromatic Hydrocarbons Contained in Marijuana Smoke on Cytochrome P450 2C9 Activity. Drug Metabolism and Pharmacokinetics. 2012;27(3): 294-300. Doi: https://doi.org/10.2133/dmpk.DMPK-11-RG-107.

14. Yamaori S, Okamoto Y, Yamamoto I, Watanabe K. Cannabidiol, a major phytocannabinoid, as a potent atypical inhibitor for CYP2D6. Drug Metabolism and Disposition: The Biological Fate of Chemicals. 2011;39(11):2049-2056. Doi: https://doi.org/10.1124/dmd.111.041384.

15. Stout S, Cimino N. Exogenous cannabinoids as substrates, inhibitors, and inducers of human drug metabolizing enzymes: A systematic review. Drug Metabolism Reviews. 2014;46(1):86-95. Doi: https://doi.org/10.3109/

03602532.2013.849268.

16. Watanabe K, Yamaori S, Funahashi T, Kimura T, & Yamamoto I. Cytochrome P450 enzymes involved in the metabolism of tetrahydrocannabinols and cannabinol by human hepatic microsomes. Life Sciences. 2007;80(15):1415-1419. Doi: https://doi.org/10.1016/j.lfs.2006.12.032.

17 Geffrey A, Pollack S, Bruno P, Thiele E. Drug–drug interaction between clobazam and cannabidiol in children with refractory epilepsy. Epilepsia. 2015;56(8):1246-1251. Doi: https://doi.org/10.1111/epi.13060.

Section 5 | Patient Care

1. Maccallum CA, Russo EB. Practical considerations in medical cannabis administration and dosing. European Journal of Internal Medicine. 2018;49:12-19. Doi: https://doi.org/10.1016/j.ejim.2018.01.004.

2. Therapeutic Goods Administration. Medicinal cannabis - guidance documents. 2018. Available at: https://www.tga.gov.au/medicinal-cannabis-guidance-documents. Accessed on 28 March 2018.

3. Ben-Shabat S, Fride E, Sheskin T, et al. An entourage effect: Inactive endogenous fatty acid glycerol esters enhance 2-arachidonoyl-glycerol cannabinoid activity. European Journal of Pharmacology. 1998;353(1):23-31. Doi: https://doi.org/10.1016/S0014-2999(98)00392-6.

4. Therapeutic Goods Administration. Guidance for the use of medicinal cannabis in Australia: Overview. 2017. Available at: https://www.tga.gov.au/publication/guidance-use-medicinal-cannabis-australia-overview. Accessed on 28 March 2018.

5. Project CBD. Cannabis Dosing. Available at: https://www.projectcbd.org/guidance/cannabis-dosing. Accessed March 28, 2018.

6. Tambaro S, Bortolato M. Cannabinoid-related agents in the treatment of anxiety disorders: current knowledge and future perspectives. Recent Patents on CNS Drug Discovery. 2012;7(1):25-40. Available at: https://www.ncbi.nlm.nih.gov/pmc/articles/PMC3691841/.

7. Otten R, Engels RC. Testing bidirectional effects between cannabis use and depressive symptoms: moderation by the serotonin transporter gene. Addict Biol. 2013 Sep;18(5):826-35. doi: 10.1111/j.1369-1600.2011.00380.x.

8. Zettl U, Rommer P, Hipp P, Patejdl R. Evidence for the efficacy and effectiveness of THC-CBD oromucosal spray in symptom management of patients with spasticity due to multiple sclerosis. Therapeutic Advances in Neurological Disorders. 2016;9(1):9-30. doi: https://doi.

org/10.1177/1756285615612659.

9. Sachse-Seeboth C, Pfeil J, Sehrt D, Meineke I, Tzvetkov M, Bruns E, Poser W, Vormfelde SV, Brockmöller J. Interindividual variation in the pharmacokinetics of Delta9-tetrahydrocannabinol as related to genetic polymorphisms in CYP2C9. Clin Pharmacol Ther. 2009 Mar;85(3):273-6. doi: 10.1038/clpt.2008.213.

10. Bland TM, Haining RL, Tracy TS, Callery PS. CYP2C-catalyzed delta9-tetrahydrocannabinol metabolism: kinetics, pharmacogenetics and interaction with phenytoin. Biochem Pharmacol. 2005 Oct 1;70(7):1096-103. doi: 10.1016/j.bcp.2005.07.007

11. Stout S, Cimino N. Exogenous cannabinoids as substrates, inhibitors, and inducers of human drug metabolizing enzymes: A systematic review. Drug Metabolism Reviews. 2014;46(1):86-95. Doi: https://doi.org/10.3109/03602532.2013.849268.

Section 6 | Delivery Methods

1. Maccallum CA, Russo EB. Practical considerations in medical cannabis administration and dosing. European Journal of Internal Medicine. 2018;49:12-19. Doi: https://doi.org/10.1016/j.ejim.2018.01.004.

2. Therapeutic Goods Administration. Guidance for the use of medicinal cannabis in Australia: Overview. 2017. Available at: https://www.tga.gov.au/publication/guidance-use-medicinal-cannabis-australia-overview. Accessed on 28 March 2018.

3. Huestis MA. Human cannabinoid pharmacokinetics. Chem Biodivers. 2007;4(8):1770–1804. doi:10.1002/cbdv.200790152

4. Syqe Medical. Syqe InhalerTM. https://www.syqemedical.com/. Published 2017.

5. McGilveray IJ. Pharmacokinetics of cannabinoids. Pain Res Manag. 2005 Autumn;10 Suppl A:15A-22A. https://www.ncbi.nlm.nih.gov/pubmed/16237477

6. Ardent. Direct Sublingual THC Dosing – The New Frontier of Cannabis Administration. https://ardentcannabis.com/sublingual-thc/. Published 11 Aug 2018.

7. Medical Jane. Consumption Methods. https://www.medicaljane.com/category/cannabis-classroom/consuming-cannabis/. Updated 2019.

8. Hammell D, Zhang L, Ma F, et al. Transdermal cannabidiol reduces inflammation and pain☐ related behaviours in a rat model of arthritis. European Journal of Pain. 2016;20(6):936-948. doi: https://doi.org/10.1002/ejp.818.

9. Cannapedia. Rectal Cannabis Suppositories. 2015. Available at: http://

www.cannapedia.cz/en/cannabis-treatment-instructions-and-manuals/
rectal-cannabis-suppositories. Accessed April 5, 2018.
10. Huestis, M. Human Cannabinoid Pharmacokinetics. Chemistry
& Biodiversity. 2007;4(8):1770-1804. Doi: https://doi.org/10.1002/
cbdv.200790152.
11. Hasan I, Zulkifle M, Ansari A.H., Sherwani A.M.K., Shakir M. History
of Ancient Egyptian Obstetrics & Gynecology: A Review. J. Microbiol.
Biotech. Res. 2011, 1 (1): 35-39. https://www.jmbronline.com/index.php/
JMBR/article/view/5/5
12. Courtney W. Achimia. Dr. Courtney's raw cannabis juice. https://www.
alchimiaweb.com/blogen/dr-courtneys-raw-cannabis-juice/. 2014.

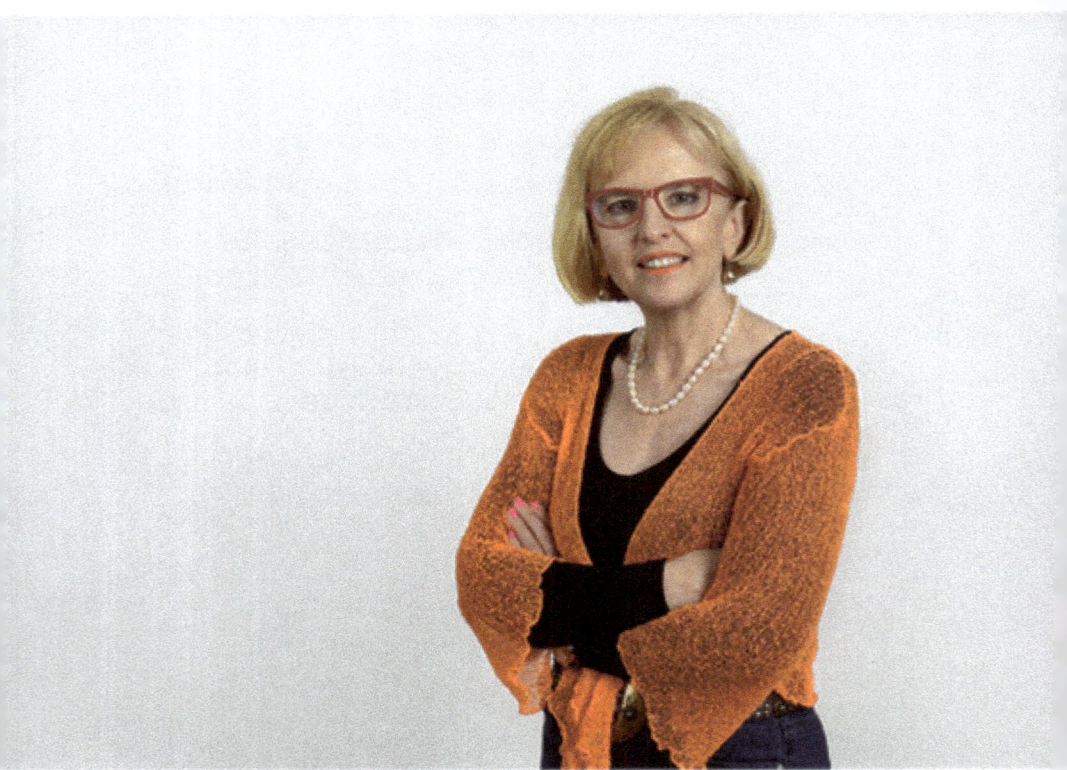

Thank you for reading my book. I hope you enjoyed it and are inspired to explore this remarkable whole plant medicine.

Your feedback is highly appreciated, please send any comments to info@medihuanna.com

Kind Regards

Dr Teresa Towpik

www.ingramcontent.com/pod-product-compliance
Lightning Source LLC
Chambersburg PA
CBHW041259040426
42334CB00028BA/3086